THE BATTERED CHILD SYNDROME

AF740201

To
May, Benjamin and Michelle

THE BATTERED CHILD SYNDROME

SELWYN M. SMITH B.S. (Sydney)
M.D. Hons (Birmingham)
M.R.C., Psych., D.P.M. (London)

Associate Professor of Psychiatry, University of Ottawa, and Head, Forensic Department, Royal Ottawa Hospital, Ottawa, Ontario.

Foreword by

Professor KEITH SIMPSON C.B.E., M.A. (Oxon) M.D., F.R.C.P., F.R.C.Path.

Home Office Pathologist and University Professor of Forensic Medicine, London

BUTTERWORTHS

LONDON · BOSTON

Sydney · Wellington · Durban · Toronto

362
.7
SMI

THE BUTTERWORTH GROUP

ENGLAND

Butterworth & Co (Publishers) Ltd
London: 88 Kingsway, WC2B 6AB

AUSTRALIA

Butterworths Pty Ltd
Sydney: 586 Pacific Highway, NSW 2067
Melbourne: 343 Little Collins Street, 3000
Brisbane: Commonwealth Bank Building,
King George Square, 4000

SOUTH AFRICA

Butterworth & Co (South Africa) (Pty) Ltd
Durban: 152–154 Gale Street

NEW ZEALAND

Butterworths of New Zealand Ltd
Wellington: 26–28 Waring Taylor Street, 1

CANADA

Butterworth & Co (Canada) Ltd
Toronto: 2265 Midland Avenue,
Scarborough, Ontario, M1P 4S1

USA

Butterworths (Publishers) Inc
161 Ash Street,
Reading, Mass. 01867

All rights reserved. No part of this publication may be reproduced or transmitted in any form or by any means, including photocopying and recording, without the written permission of the copyright holder, application for which should be addressed to the publisher. Such written permission must also be obtained before any part of this publication is stored in a retrieval system of any nature.

This book is sold subject to the Standard Conditions of Sale of Net Books and may not be re-sold in the UK below the net price given by the Publishers in their current price list.

First published 1975

ISBN 0 407 00046 1

© Butterworth & Co (Publishers) Ltd 1975

LEICESTER UNIVERSITY LIBRARY

Withdrawn from University Leicester Library

5.4.76

2010293354

Library of Congress Cataloging in Publication Data

Smith, Selwyn M
The battered child syndrome.

Bibliography: p.
Includes index.
1. Cruelty to children. 2. Infanticide.
I. Title. [DNLM: 1. Child abuse. WA320 S659b]
HV713. S6 364.1'5 75-26150
ISBN 0-407-00046-1

Text set in 10/11 pt. IBM Journal, printed by photolithography, and bound in Great Britain at The Pitman Press, Bath

Contents

Part III

PSYCHIATRIC, PSYCHOLOGICAL AND SOCIAL CHARACTERISTICS OF THE PARENTS

Part IV

INTERPRETATION OF THE FINDINGS

APPENDICES

Foreword

The very serious nature of the problem of the ill-treated child has become unfolded all too slowly for those with a conscience that was troubled by the writings of Silverman, Wooley and Evans, Kempe and others in the 1950s. Neither the Memorandum of the British Paediatric Society, nor the N.S.P.C.C. survey did much to enquire into the fundamental causes of the problem, and though doctors, nurses, pathologists and the police became aware of the need to recognize it – and more practised in doing so – no effective impact was made on social, psychiatric and health workers, on magistrates and lawyers to ensure better handling of offenders: too little was known of the socio-psychiatric background to enable the Courts to handle such cases wisely. Tragedies like Maria Colwell that 'should never have happened' slipped all too easily through the preventive nets, and suspended sentences, like deferred decisions, sometimes proved fatal.

Selwyn Smith has, in this new work, explored the unknowns in the background of battered baby cases in a scholarly, yet thoroughly practical, clinical study that will undoubtedly make this book a classic in this field of paediatrics and socio-psychiatry. It does what Steele and Pollock set out to do in Kempe's 'master-guide' so much more thoroughly and penetratingly, dissecting out the tangled causes of ill-feeling and baby bashing, love–hate relationships and frustration that ends in such tragic hurt to children with a clarity that must lead to better understanding – and treatment, if not of prevention.

It is a pleasure to read such good writing, to savour another sample of the quality of work that has brought so much repute to English medicine, and to feel Selwyn Smith's deep concern and sympathy for parents and others who drift into handling children in a way no society can tolerate. Shaftesbury and Barnardo had the same understanding, and their percipience of the needs of neglected children created great changes in attitude, and improvement in living conditions and prospects for children. Selwyn Smith's new study may well do the same.

K. S.

Preface

Nearly a century ago, Samuel West the founder of Great Ormond Street Children's Hospital observed and recorded the salient features of what is now called the battered child syndrome. He noted the very tender age of the child (5 weeks), the main symptoms (unexplained painful swelling of an arm), their recurrent nature (there had been previous similar, asymmetrical lesions in the other arm and leg), the delay in bringing the child to hospital, and the prevalence of the condition in other children of the family (three other children irrespective of sex had been similarly affected when they were babies and two of their cousins also had swellings of the arms or legs at similar ages). He also observed the traumatic nature of the symptoms ('greenstick' features) and commented that the lesions resolved when the children were in hospital. However, he did not state the origin of the violence but demonstrated another important feature of the syndrome – the reluctance of observers to enquire into how the trauma happened.

The coining of the dramatic name for the syndrome by Kempe in 1962 has served useful in rivetting the attention of a reluctant public to the hard realities of the situation. However, as is often the case with issues ranking high in public interest, systematic information on baby battering continues to be scarce. Many claims concerning the nature and scope of the phenomenon are based on isolated observations and on local, uncontrolled clinical studies. This lack of information has been commented on by Norman Polansky (1968).

> 'Our ignorance regarding the problems of child abuse and child neglect is, in the year 1968, not quite total, but it is severe enough to be inexcusable. We do *not* know what the incidence *nor* prevalence of these

> conditions are. We do not know how to go about casefinding and/or identification of these conditions. We have little knowledge of how to discriminate levels of severity, and are poor at prognosticating future course, with or without available treatments, in many instances. Finally we do not know how to "treat" either of these social conditions in the sense of bringing about enduring change in the parents involved with much consistency, and with any efficiency. Other than that, we are scientifically in an excellent position'.

The aim of this book has been to improve the lack of systematic knowledge by bringing together the published professional opinions on the characteristics of the parents and children involved so that systematic testing of hypotheses can be carried out. The book also provides a comprehensive report of a broadly based research study that was conducted from the Department of Psychiatry, University of Birmingham between 1970 and 1974. Many of the findings reported from the study are at variance with the American experience of the phenomenon. It is hoped that such differences will stimulate the impetus for further research into the subject.

So many people have helped me in the planning, collection and analysis of the data that it would take several pages to do justice to their contributions. I would like to record my gratitude to Mrs. Ruth Hanson, for her assistance with the research, design, psychological testing and statistics, and Mrs. Sheila Noble for her untiring efforts in obtaining the social data. Mrs. Irene Brown and Mrs. Margaret Hall and the staff of the Hospital Statistics Department provided ready help with computer programming. Dr. Leo Honingsberger and Dr. Graham Harding undertook and read the EEGs. Dr. Roy Astley and Dr. Keith Tonge interpreted the x-rays and Assistant Chief Constable Harry Robinson helped with the Criminal Records. Mrs. Sue Knight competently typed the manuscript and Miss Pat Pottie read the proofs.

The impetus to this research study was provided by Professor William Trethowan, and Dr. John Varley who also provided wise counsel throughout the vicissitudes of implementation. Mr. Paul Cadbury and Mr. Anthony Wilson and other members of the Steering Committee were generous with encouragement, advice and guidance. The interest and co-operation of the medical and nursing staff of Birmingham Children's Hospital and other hospitals made the completion of the study possible. Generous financial support for the study was provided by the Endowment Fund of the United Birmingham Hospitals and the Barrow and Geraldine S. Cadbury Trust.

Gratitude is also due to Mrs. Lorna Seager and her staff of the Barnes Medical Library who obtained many of the references cited in this book, and to Mr. David Drury and his staff of the Department of Medical Illustration, Birmingham Children's Hospital who photographed the children and designed many of the illustrations. Mr. Keith Rogers of the Television and Film Unit of Birmingham University designed the dust jacket. Some short passages from this book have already appeared in articles in the *British Medical Journal, British Journal of Psychiatry, New Society* and *Journal of the Royal Society of Health*, to all of which I would like to make due acknowledgement. I am also grateful to Lund Humphries Publishers Ltd who have kindly granted permission to reproduce their illustrations (*Figures 1* and *4*).

Finally, special gratitude is due to my parents who accepted an undue measure of neglect while I pursued the study and to my wife May, for sharing all the hopes, frustrations and detail surrounding the writing of this book. To her, my greatest debt is due.

S.M.S.

Tables

Figures

COLOUR PLATES

(The colour plate section appears facing page 140)

PART I

BACKGROUND TO THE PROBLEM: A REVIEW OF THE MEDICAL, SOCIAL AND LEGAL LITERATURE

Chapter 1

Maltreatment of Children: An Historical Perspective

INTRODUCTION

Over the centuries children have been killed, maimed, starved, abandoned, neglected and chastised with cruelty. Despite this the maltreatment of children by their parents has only aroused public concern in recent times. This delay in recognition is to be wondered at; as is the phenomenon of maltreatment itself. It is the purpose of this chapter to examine briefly the historical background of each of these inhuman acts and some of the reasons for society's indifference to such tragic events. Several authors (Garrison, 1965; Radbill, 1968; Bakan, 1971; Resnick, 1972) have provided excellent accounts of various aspects of the history of child abuse and have provided the main sources of references to this chapter.

MOTIVES

The killing of children goes back as far as recorded history and the motives given for this act are many (Radbill, 1968; Resnick, 1972). In Papua and in Cochin China infanticide was an acceptable method of family planning and a mother was despised and likened to an animal if she had too many children. In some cultures a limit of three children per family was set and those born after the third were killed. The dishonour of bearing an illegitimate child was another primary cause of infanticide, particularly prevalent among the Arabs who killed their young girls. In polygamous societies there was a taboo which kept the mother away from the embraces of her husband during the lactation period; a time when infants were especially at risk.

Greed for money was another motive which led to infanticide. Eighty per cent of the illegitimate children put out to nurse in London during the nineteenth century died, for unscrupulous nurses collected their fees and then promptly did away with the babies. Edwin Chadwick called attention to the insurance system of 'burial clubs'; for an investment of about one pound, three to five pounds could be realized when a child was buried. Unscrupulous and greedy midwives were also a threat to the infant's life for they would sometimes accept fees to 'arrange for' the death of the newborn infant.

The twins Romulus and Remus were the classical examples of the motives of greed for power. When Kings feared their replacement, elimination of the newborn heir would be carried out. When Pharoah feared the Jews, he ordered the slaughter of the innocent newborn males (Exodus, 1:9) and when Herod feared the coming of a Messiah he ordered the slaying of all children in Bethlehem (Matthew, 2:16) (*see Figure 1*).

Twins, monstrous births or congenitally defective children were feared by man as they frequently foreshadowed evil (Radbill, 1968). In China, India and throughout the Orient, deformed children were usually destroyed at birth. The Greeks and Romans killed their weak and deformed infants in the superstitious hope that only the strong would survive. Plato, Aristotle and other philosophers lectured that survival of the fittest was necessary to strengthen the race and this belief was incorporated into the Roman Law of the Twelve Tables which forebade rearing deformed children. During the period of the Caesars, infanticide – always legal in Rome – received the approval of philosophers like Seneca (Bakan, 1971). Morals decayed, broken marriages became common and exposure of infants frequent. Athenian children were also at risk for if a Council of Spartan elders judged a child to be weak or deformed it was cast from a mountain into a deep canyon.

Ritual sacrifice accounted for countless infant deaths. Hecate, a Greek God to whom sacrifices were made at the crossroads, was called Infanticida when she demanded children (Benét, 1965). In certain fertility rites in China, India, Mexico and Peru, children were cast into rivers as offerings to water gods in order that good harvests would follow. The Bible also contains many allusions to ritual sacrifice (*see Figure 2*). Solomon 'did . . . build a high place for Chemosh . . . and for Molech' (1 Kings 11:7), gods to whom children were sacrificed by burning. King Ahaz 'burnt his children in the fire' (2 Chronicles 33:6). Superstitions also accounted for the belief that slain infants would benefit the sterile woman, cure disease and confer health, vigour,

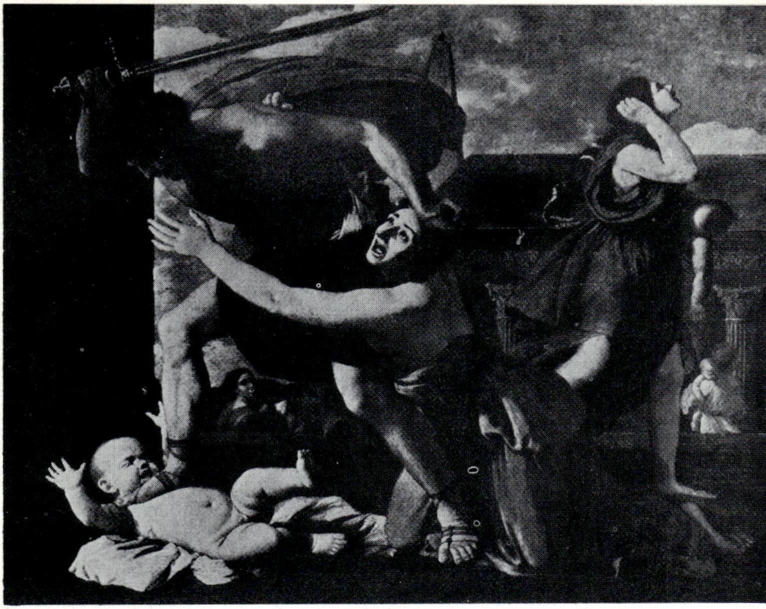

Figure 1. Massacre of the Innocents by Nicholas Poussin

and youthfulness. Mothers were fed the flesh of slain infants to produce strong offspring and the flesh was also fed to favoured siblings to make them strong and healthy.

To ensure durability of important buildings children were sometimes buried under the foundations (Bakan, 1971). In Germany during the sixteenth century children were buried alive beneath the doorsteps of public buildings (Dunn, 1920) and in the seventeenth century children were immured in the dikes of Oldenburg (Stern, 1948).

The practice of immurement of children in the foundations of erected structures has an ancient history. Joshua's curse (Joshua 6:26) against anyone who rebuilt Jericho – 'he shall lay the foundations thereof in his first born and in his youngest son shall he set up the gates of it' – was indeed fulfilled against Hiel the Bethelite (1 Kings 16:34), if the Biblical account is historically accurate. Archeological discoveries of jars of bones of newborn infants under buildings have confirmed how widespread this practice was (Potter, 1949). As late as 1873 female infanticide was permitted in China. 'It was and may still be the custom

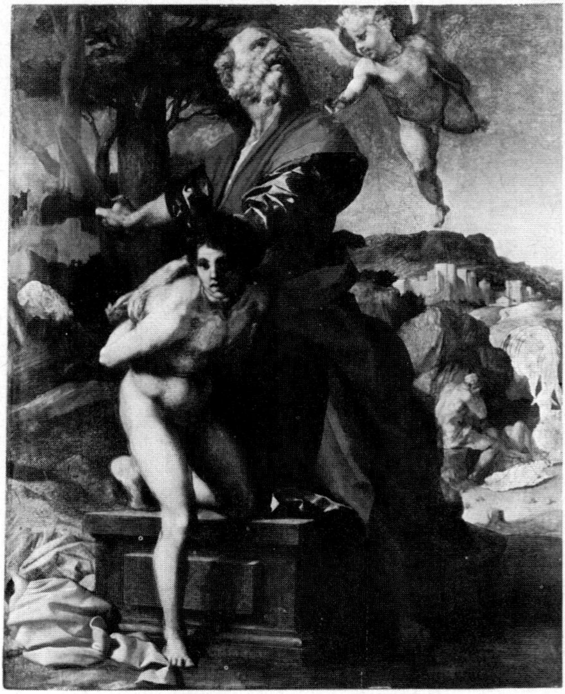

Figure 2. Sacrifice of Isaac by Andrea del Sarto
(Reproduced by permission of
The Cleveland Museum of Art,
Delia E. and L. E. Holden Funds.)

for new pottery furnaces in the Kiang-si province to be consecrated with the secret shedding of children's blood'. (Stern, 1948).

Sumner was one of the first modern sociologists to recognize that the killing of children has been a significant feature of human social history.

> 'Child sacrifice has been a significant feature of human social history and expresses the deepest horror and suffering produced by the experience of the human lot. Men must do it. Their interests demand it, however much it might pain them. Human sacrifice may be said to have been universal. It lasted down to the half-civilized stage of all nations and has barely ceased among the present half-civilized peoples.'
>
> (Sumner, 1906)

LITERARY REFERENCES

The ubiquity of infanticide in European thought is evident in Goethe's use of the theme in Faust, for Gretchen who has borne Faust a child later drowns it. Werner (1917) commenting on the background which may have led Goethe to include this infanticide episode in his drama concluded that no single event influenced Goethe – 'the fact is that infanticide was so common in the last half of the eighteenth century that no one can be looked upon as the sole source of any particular literary production'.

Other literary sources bear testimony to this widespread practice. In Europe in 1781 a contest was held for the best essay on how to prevent infanticide. 'The prize question how infanticide might be checked, has alarmed so many scholars in all the faculties that one is amazed at the large number of essays submitted' (quoted in Werner, 1917). Johann Pestalozzi, a distinguished educator, in his essay discussed 15 cases in one chapter.

> 'Infanticide! Do I dream or am I awake! Is it possible, this deed? Does it happen? Does the unnamed happen? No, not the unnamed, the named, the crime which has found expression in words. Conceal thy face, O Century! Bow down O Europe! From the seats of justice comes the answer: my children are killed by the thousands at the hands of those who gave birth to them. In vain runs the blood of thy infanticides, O Europe! Let thy rulers remove the causes of their despair, and thou wilt save their children. . . .'
>
> (quoted in Werner, 1917)

Frederick the Great, King of Prussia between 1740 and 1786, particularly concerned himself with the problems of infanticide and abolished church penance for unmarried mothers because the punishment and disgrace 'give occasion to infanticide' (quoted in Werner, 1917). In England the relationship between illegitimacy and infanticide was the theme of the popular ballad '*The Cruel Mother*'.

> 'She leaned herself against a thorn,
> there she had two pretty babes born.
> Then she cut her topknot from her head,
> and tied those babies hands and legs.
> She took her penknife keen and sharp,
> and pierced those babies tender hearts.
> She buried them under a marble stone,
> and then she said she would go home . . .' (quoted in Bronson, 1959)

Shakespeare was profoundly aware of the infanticidal impulse. He has Lady Macbeth say:

> 'I have given suck and know,
> How tender 'tis to love the babe that milks me;

I would while it was smiling in my face
Have pluck'd my nipple from his boneless gums,
And dash'd the brains out. . . .'

(*Macbeth,* Act I, Scene VII)

Another example of how the infanticidal impulse may be triggered is given in *King John.*

Salisbury: 'His passion is so ripe it needs must break.'
Pembroke: 'And when it breaks, I fear will issue thence,
The foul corruption of a sweet child's death.'

(*King John,* Act IV, Scene II)

Writing in 1845, Benjamin Disraeli, in his novel *Sybil,* gives a harrowing description of the early life of a child, who grew up unknown, and was given the name of Devilsdust. 'Infanticide', he wrote, 'is practised as extensively and legally in England as it is on the banks of the Ganges'.

Freud (1950) argued that everyone 'possesses in his unconscious an instrument by which he can interpret the expressions of the unconscious of another', and this observation may certainly apply to children. Adler (1951) has observed that many children are particularly afraid of being struck. Bakan (1971) has argued that:

> 'In some way, the child who is hated registers that possibility somewhere in the recesses of his mind. Yet his immaturity stands in the way of his apprehending it; and the wisdom of psychological inheritance provides him with innocence which is at once also a protection'.

A crack in the innocence of both adults and children exists in the poems and stories adults recite for the entertainment of children. It is interesting to observe that some of the most popular children's folklore in Western culture are infanticidal in content. To cite just a few: 'Hush a Bye Baby', 'Humpty Dumpty', 'Jack and the Beanstalk', 'Hansel and Gretel', 'The Pied Piper of Hamelin', 'Snow White and the Seven Dwarfs', and 'Punch and Judy'. Bakan (1971) believes that:

> 'The deepest wishes and concerns of people find their way into fiction and myth, while that same fiction and myth provide them with entertainment. Hard thoughts, thoughts which would otherwise be too unpleasant to think, smuggle their way into these fanciful renditions. There they are held fast in a frame of unbelief. Some things are simply too terrible to think about if one believes them. Thus one does not believe them in order to make it possible to think about them.'

It is thus paradoxical, if Bakan's argument is accepted, that disguising infanticide and child cruelty in a wrap of untruth allows the truth to be conveyed and revealed.

The background to the story of '*Le Petit Poucet*' which in English has become the story of '*Hop o' my Thumb*' has been clearly described by Iona and Peter Opie in their book *The Classic Fairy Tales* (Opie and Opie, 1974). The name 'Hop o' my Thumb' (Hop on my Thumb) was the term for a tiny person which was in common use 400 years ago. The deliberate abandonment of children whom the parents are no longer able to support is, of course, an old theme, not only in fiction. The trick Little Poucet plays on the ogre, to good effect, swapping the crowns of gold worn by the ogre's children while they sleep for the common bonnets worn by his brothers, so that the ogre in his drunken stupor slaughters his own seven children (*see Figure 3*), also has counterparts. (It is interesting to note that the masterly but horrific

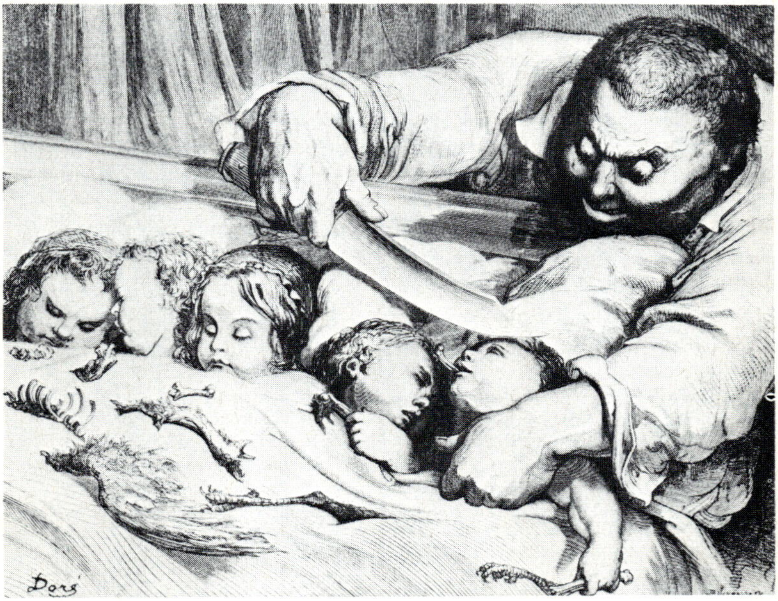

Figure 3. The ogre about to cut the throats of his seven daughters. The horrific illustration by Gustave Dore of the story of Hop o' my Thumb

(Reproduced by courtesy of the British Library; copyright George Rainbird Ltd., photographed by John Freeman.)

illustration by Gustave Doré (*see Figure 3*) which appeared in *Les Contes de Perrault*, 1862, was suppressed in the English edition.) In the Hessian story of '*Sweetheart Roland*', collected by the Grimm brothers, a witch executes her own daughter instead of her step-daughter, due to the heroine changing her place in the bed while the other girl sleeps; and in the Swedish story of *Roll*, a giant kills his own eight daughters because Roll, in the night, has switched their caps for his brothers' headcloths. The second century mythographer Hyginus tells the story of Themisto, wife of Athamas, whose hatred of her rival Ino was such that she determined to destroy her children. She instructed the nurse to dress Ino's children in black nightgowns, and her own children in white, so that she might differentiate between them in the night. But she was unaware the nurse was Ino in disguise, and Ino put the white nightgowns on her own children and the black on Themisto's. In the dusk the children Themisto murders are her own. There are other variations on the same theme told in other countries (Opie and Opie, 1974).

The acute situation concerning children in Eighteenth Century Britain, is ironically described by Jonathan Swift who urged 'the mother to let them suck plentifully, so as to render them plump and fat for a good table'. The advantages of fattening and then eating children, was that it would prevent 'that horrible practice of women murdering their bastard children, alas! too frequent among us, sacrificing the poor innocent babes . . . more to avoid the expense than the shame' (quoted in Eddy, 1965).

Though Malthus published his essay discussing 'poverty and misery arising from a too rapid increase of population', in 1798, he failed to argue convincingly against infanticide as a method of population control. This fact was pointed out by Charles Darwin who was aware that infanticide was a harsh and widespread reality.

> '(Malthus) has discussed these several checks, but he does not lay stress enough on what is probably the most important of all, namely infanticide, and the habit of procuring abortion. These practices now prevail in many quarters of the world; and infanticide seems formerly to have prevailed, on a still more extensive scale. These practices appear to have originated in savages, recognizing the difficulty, or rather impossibility, of supporting all the infants that are born.'
>
> (Darwin, 1936)

Public awareness about infanticide accompanied the growth of large urban-industrial centres in the late nineteenth and early twentieth centuries. The situation is manifested by the following summary from an 1890 edition of the *Encyclopaedia Britannica*.

> 'The modern crime of infanticide shows no symptoms of diminishing in the leading nations of Europe. In all of them it is closely connected with illegitimacy in the class of farm and domestic servants. The crime is generally committed by the mother for the purpose of completing the concealment of her shame, and in other cases, where shame has not survived, in order to escape the burden of her child's support. The paramour sometimes aids in the crimes, which is not confined to unmarried mothers.'

The unease associated with the problem is apparent from the contradiction between the authors assignment of cause to 'illegitimacy in the class of farm and domestic servants' and his statement that crime 'is not confined to unmarried mothers'. The author goes on to describe the situation in the United Kingdom:

> 'At one time a large number of children were murdered in England for the mere purpose of obtaining the burial money from a benefit club. In 1871 the House of Commons found it necessary to appoint a select committee "to enquire as to the best means of preventing the destruction of the lives of infants put out to live by their parents . . . ". The result was the act of 1872 which provided for the compulsory registration of all houses in which more than one child under one year were received for a longer period than twenty four hours. Offences against the Act including wilful neglect of children even in a suitable house are punished by a fine of £5 or six months imprisonment with or without hard labour.'
>
> (*Encyclopaedia Britannica, 1890*)

The apathy and indifference shown by the community towards the deprived and rejected child has been depicted by Heywood (1965). She has described how society's attitudes to such children have changed. The effectiveness of these changing attitudes in protecting children from maltreatment will be discussed later.

CHILD BATTERING AND INFANTICIDE

The overlap between child battering and infanticide is considerable (Bakan, 1971). Aptekar (1931) has argued that:

> 'Infanticide is in the wider sense of the word, primitive. It would be obscuring reality to call this trait "instinctive". It is not common to all mankind. Yet it comes so near to being inherent in the primeval parent–child relationship that one is tempted to say of it: "Here if anywhere is a bit of behaviour natural to primitive man'.

The methods used in infanticide have not changed much throughout history. Blood is rarely shed (Radbill, 1968), and head trauma, strangulation and drowning are the common methods used (Resnick, 1972). Bakan (1971) also argues that 'child abuse may be a regression to a characteristic which comes very close to being "natural" to the human condition', and believes that there is little distinction between baby battering and infanticide for 'the aim of those who abuse a child is to kill the child; the reason for abusing him or her is to be rid of him or her'. Indeed many abused children do die (Helfer and Pollock, 1968). In reaching this conclusion Bakan (1971) argues that:

> 'the very largest category of victims is very young children, the frequency of victimization being closely related to the degree of care that the age

of the child demands. Children who have been directly victimized by beatings are often also victimized by neglect . . . In many instances the parents were not interested in having a child, as manifested in the proportion of victims conceived out of wedlock.'

Support for Bakan's argument is also found in Resnick's study (1972) which showed that the great bulk of neonaticides are committed simply because the child is not wanted and that 'the most common reason for neonaticide among married women is extramarital paternity'. In discussing paternal infanticide, Resnick (1972) showed that 'Fathers are more likely to kill when there is doubt about paternity and when the progeny is viewed as a financial burden or an impediment to their career'. The significance of some of these points as they related to child battering in this study will be discussed later.

MUTILATION OF CHILDREN

Children have always been the victims of mutilation practices, the most common sites being the sex organs (Radbill, 1968). Circumcision in spite of its questionable value has been practised as a religious rite since the Stone Age and indeed is the most common operation performed today. The Bible and Shakespeare also make frequent references to castration being an acceptable procedure and the important role played by the eunuch in certain societies (Brim, 1936).

In China, foot binding of female children was carried out for cosmetic purposes and its practice has only recently been discontinued. In Africa, however, various other forms of bindings to produce fashionable configurations on the arms, legs and other parts of the body are still practised.

Cranial deformation is encountered in many different parts of the world. It has been discovered in ancient skulls in the Crimea, was mentioned by Hippocrates, was prevalent among the American Indians and is still practised in the Solomon Islands. The Indians favoured flattened heads, while the Melanesians shaped their heads into elongated cones. Although it was lovingly done, and as a rule purely for cosmetic purposes, the Viceroy Toledo (sixteenth century) in a series of regulations promulgated for the care and hygiene of infants in South America recognized it as a form of child abuse and forbade its practice (Radbill, 1968).

Uvulectomy, another curious operation, practised for generations among the Berbers of Northern Morocco was carried out soon after birth to facilitate breast feeding and speech and to ensure better health throughout life.

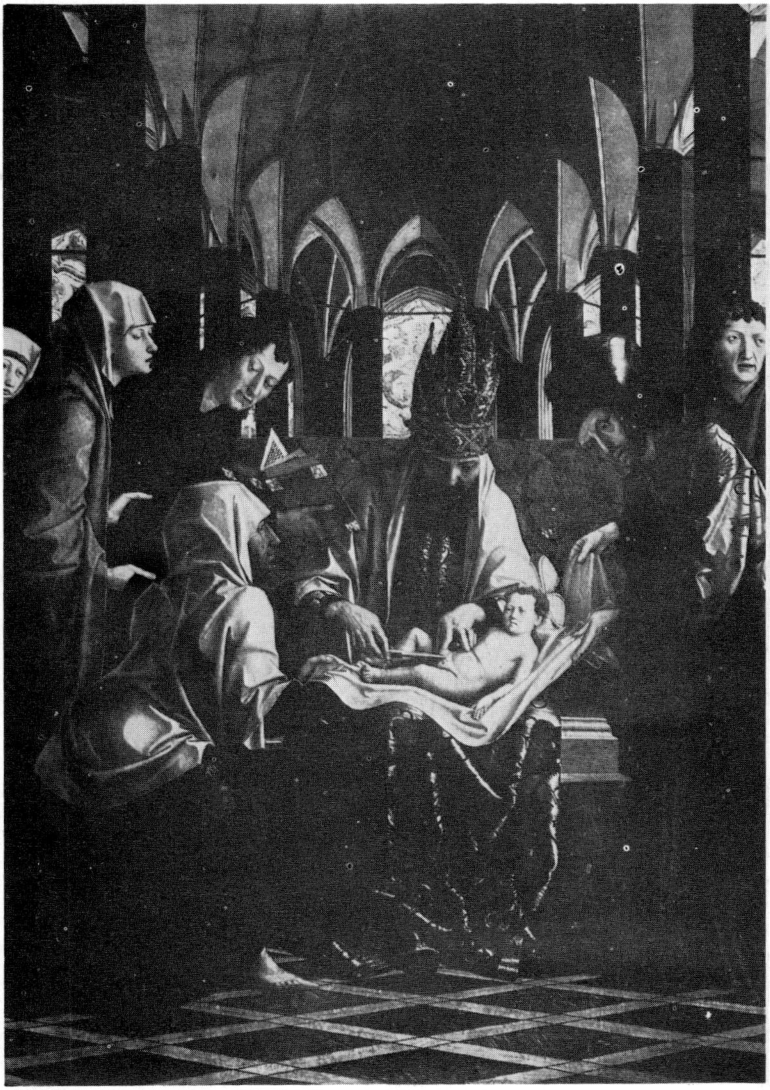

Figure 4. Circumcision of Christ (St. Wolfgang Altar Painting)

Various forms of mutilation that were clearly vicious were carried out by speculators who trafficked in children. Gouged eyes, amputated and twisted arms and legs or broken and deformed feet were inflicted upon children to arouse pity, thereby making them good beggars. Slavery was another form of abuse children often had to endure. In ancient times the rights of the father included the right to sell his child into slavery (Bakan, 1971). Girls were sold to be raised as prostitutes and boys were sold to work.

ABANDONMENT OF CHILDREN

Legend and myth have dramatized abandonment of infants from ancient times. Many famous characters in history began their lives as foundlings – Moses, Romulus and Remus, Saragon I, and Horus – to cite but a few. In Imperial Rome at the height of its moral decadence the favourite place for exposure was in the market place, where nursing mothers gathered to be hired out as wet nurses or to employ wet nurses for their own children. The rescued infants could be adopted but were more often raised in slavery or used as piteous beggars after being deformed by speculators in the baby market (Radbill, 1968).

Foundlings were especially numerous in times of war or social upheaval. From the earliest days of Christianity, institutions were founded by the Church for these unbaptized waifs. During the crusades fervent zealots left a trail of foundlings all along the course of their pilgrimages to the Holy Land. Pope Innocent III, in about 1200, encouraged institutional care for these foundlings to discourage infanticide and the Hospital of the Holy Ghost and the Order of the Holy Ghost, were assiduously devoted to the welfare of foundlings. During the reign of Louis XIII when poverty-stricken hordes inhabited Paris the frightful number of slaughtered infants induced St. Vincent de Paul to act on behalf of foundling institutions. In Russia, Catherine II, moved by the plight of abandoned children, built a foundling hospital. A basket with warm clothes was ready outside the hospital day and night to receive babies, and no questions were asked. Later the famous 'tour' or turning box was introduced to conceal the identity of the mother and spare her from shame and harassment. During the French Revolution the 'tour' was discontinued in France but was re-instated by Napoleon who also recalled the Sisters of Charity in order that they could care for the foundlings, because he wanted to save as many children as possible for the armies of France (Radbill, 1968).

The incident which led to the founding of the New York Nursery and Children's Hospital in 1854 is cited by Radbill (1968) and highlights the situation which existed at the time when the practice was for mothers to employ wet nurses for their own children.

> 'A midwife called upon a known wealthy lady whom she had attended at childbirth, and while looking at the baby, was surprised to find the infant's wet nurse in tears. Inquiry revealed that the wet nurse's child had been turned over to a foster mother. The midwife went to see the wet nurse's child and found the foster mother sick in bed in a small, dirty basement room. The foster mother's own child was dead of smallpox and the wretched squalid infant of the wet nurse was under the bed in a basket of soiled clothes'.

INDUSTRIALIZATION AND CHILD ABUSE

Urbanization and the machine age led to other forms of child abuse and increasing child mortality. Royston Pike (1966) has described in particularly vivid detail the harsh conditions which prevailed at the time of the Industrial Revolution. Though children had always worked, the advent of the machine led to their virtual enslavement for they were subjected to terrible inhumanities under the factory system. Children from 5 years of age and upward worked 16 hours a day, sometimes with irons riveted around their ankles to keep them from running away. They were starved, beaten, and in many other ways maltreated. Many succumbed to occupational diseases, and some committed suicide; few survived for any length of time. Chimney sweeping was particularly hazardous work for children. Working night and day, their efforts were usually hastened by their master burning straw behind them; they were subjected to all kinds of brutality. 'People were callous to their sufferings and when a certain woman, touched by an accident that occurred to one small sweep in her own home, befriended them as a class, her kindness was suspect' (Radbill, 1968). These children quickly deteriorated both mentally and physically. Percival Pott described cancer of the scrotum which developed among the chimney sweeps in 1775 and other children rapidly succumbed to the ravages of pulmonary consumption.

In 1802 the first Factory Act was passed in Parliament. Child labour reform initiated by Robert Owen and Sir Robert Peel broke up the pauper apprentice-system and led to the abolishment of the practice of sending boys up chimneys. The traditional rights of parents over their children persisted, however, and the Act did not apply to children under the supervision of their parents. Children who went to the mills with their parents' consent still had to work 12 hours a day and were often brutally whipped with leather thongs by tyrannical supervisors. Dipping children head first into cisterns of cold water to keep them awake was still common practice (Royston Pike, 1966).

Over a period of more than 40 years the deprived conditions of these children received the attention of Parliament. The reports and minutes of the successive committees of enquiry are extensively quoted by Royston Pike and portray the indifference many people shared towards these children's plight.

HARSH DISCIPLINE OF CHILDREN

Maltreatment of children has been justified for centuries by the belief that severe physical punishment was necessary to maintain discipline, to transmit educational ideas, to please certain gods or to expel evil spirits (Radbill, 1968). Whipping children has been the prerogative of teachers as well as of parents, who often justified their action by quoting the Biblical aphorism 'He that spareth the rod hateth his son' (Proverbs, XIII, 24). In the schools of Sumer, 5000 years ago, there was 'a man in charge of the whip' to punish boys upon the slightest pretext (Kramer, 1956).

There was a time in most Christian centuries when children were whipped on Innocents Day to commemorate the slaughter of the innocents of Herod. Beatings to drive out the devil were of a form of psychiatric treatment especially applicable to children, and where epilepsy was attributed to demoniacal possession, the sufferer was thrashed soundly to expel the demon. In India there was a sacred iron chain expressly for this purpose.

Ancient philosophers beat their pupils unmercifully. Parents, teachers and ministers alike believed that the only cure for the 'foolishness bound up in the heart of the child' was repression by use of the rod. The ferule was used by Roman schoolmasters as the instrument for punishment. In England and America, pictures of pedagogues usually showed them armed with a birch. Michael Udall, headmaster at Eton during the reign of Elizabeth I, was noted for his addiction to the use of four apple twigs.

It was taken for granted that parents and guardians had every right to treat their children as they saw fit. Pepys beat his boy until he (Pepys) was out of breath; John Wesley, Frederick the Great, Lady Jane Gray and many other famous figures complained bitterly about their treatment in childhood. King Henry VI was regularly flogged as a child, and though he became a scholar and a gentleman he was a most unhappy individual (Godfrey, 1907). Charles I was more fortunate for he had Mungo Murray available as a whipping boy to substitute for him when punishment was indicated. The German-born Queen Caroline complained that the English were not well bred because they were not whipped enough when they were young. Lady Abergane beat her own child in a fit of passion and when the father complained she threw the child so violently to the ground that his skull was fractured and he was killed (Godfrey, 1907).

History also reveals that there were influential personages who spoke out against the maltreatment of children. Plato in 400 B.C. advised teachers 'to train children not by compulsion but as if they were playing' and Plutarch 300 years later decried the use of the whip (Radbill, 1968). The calvinistic view that children were imps of darkness led Thomas Ingeland in 1570 to write a protest skit which he called '*A Prettie and Merrie New Interlude Called the Disobedient Child*', which describes a boy who 'through many stryppes was dead and cold' (quoted in Godfrey 1907). The cruelty he experienced at Eton induced Roger Ascham in 1570 to write '*The Schoolmaster*' in which he advocated love instead of fear in teaching children (Benét, 1965). John Locke a century later, pleaded for schoolmasters to reserve the rod for moral faults only.

Western education gradually began to yield to the demands of exemplars of modern thought, such as Erasmus, who although rearing his own children with harsh formality was strongly influenced by Sir Thomas More, who used peacock feathers to beat his daughters (Radbill, 1968). John Frank pioneered the establishment of legal regulations that curbed corporal punishment in schools at the end of the eighteenth century (Ariès, 1962). Pressure against child abuse was also exerted by those outside the educational system. In 1611, Roger L'Estrange published a book '*The Children's Petition*', that begged parents to show more lenience towards their children. In 1698 another book appeared entitled '*Lex Forcia, A Sensible Address to Parliament for an Act to Remedy the Foul Abuse of Children at Schools*' (Dunn, 1920). Charles Dickens in his novels also convincingly portrayed the wrongs inflicted on children by their parents in the nineteenth century. The beating scene in his autobiographical *David Copperfield* (Chapter IV) focuses sharply upon the harshness displayed towards children.

> 'He walked me up to my room slowly and gravely – I am certain he had a delight in that formal parade of executing justice – and, when we got there, suddenly twisted my head under his arm. He beat me then, as if he would have beaten me to death. Then he was gone; and the door was locked outside; and I was lying, fevered and hot and torn and sore and raging in my puny way upon the floor.'

'The Dickens' remains as a euphemism for the beating of children today.

LEGISLATION AGAINST THE MALTREATMENT OF CHILDREN

The Code of Hammurabi about 4000 years ago, provided that if a nurse allowed a suckling child to die in her hands and substituted another her breast should be amputated (Garrison, 1965). In ancient Egypt infanticide was common, but it was not legal. The Thebans made it a capital offence, and there is an Egyptian record of a child murderer who was ordered to carry the slain infant in her arms for 3 days and 3 nights (Radbill, 1968). Though the Patria Potestas gave a father supreme right to sell, mutilate or even kill his offspring as early as 700 B.C. infanticide was relatively uncommon in Ancient Rome (Bakan, 1971). The Laws of the Twelve Tables (about 450 B.C.) modified the Patria Potestas so that a son could be sold only three times. The laws of Augustus Caesar in A.D. 4 checked the Patria Potestas and indirectly aided children but the exposure of children continued unabated. Child welfare laws and agitation on behalf of children were frequent under succeeding emperors. Tiberius ordered the death penalty for Carthagenian priests who sacrificed children by fire, but the practice continued in secret. The efforts of Empress Faustina to save female infants from destruction during the second century were also short-lived for the next century was a hazardous one for children (Garrison, 1965).

The Bible and Koran prohibited infanticide. Philo Judaeus in the first century after Christ proclaimed that infanticide was a crime and in the next century Tertullian, one of the fathers of the Christian Church, in speaking of infanticide said 'murder is murder in any shape' and a sin against the commandment, 'Thou shalt not kill' (quoted in Radbill, 1968). Through the influence of Christianity, edicts against infanticide and the sale of children into slavery were issued by Constantine (A.D. 315) and Valentinian III (A.D. 451) and others. Infanticide by exposure or otherwise had been established as a crime by Barnabas in the time of the Apostles. In A.D. 305 a sentence of excommunication for life was decreed (Garrison, 1965). Sixtus and Gregory XIV in the sixteenth century and Frederick the Great in the eighteenth century issued stern edicts against infanticide.

In 1556, Henry II of France decreed death to women who concealed the birth of a child and shortly after King James I in England passed a similar law but it subsequently had to be repealed. Jean Jacques Rousseau (1712–1778) wrote, 'Let us speak less of the duties of children and more of their rights', but it is interesting to observe that he abandoned his own children (Benét, 1965). Addison in 1773 also expressed concern at the situation: 'There is scarce an assizes, where some unhappy wretch is not executed for the murder of a child. And how many more of these monsters of inhumanity may we suppose to be wholly undiscovered or cleared for want of legal evidence' (quoted in Caulfield, 1931). In 1803 an Act was passed which placed women tried for murder of illegitimate children under the same laws and penalties as those pertaining to murder.

One of the most important medicolegal contributions in the seventeenth century was Swammerdam's discovery in 1667 that foetal lungs will float in water after respiration has taken place (Radbill, 1968). This discovery solved the vexing problem of determining whether the baby was born alive before it was killed. It was first put to practical application by Johann Schreyer in the case of a peasant girl aged 15 years who was accused of infanticide in 1681; the infants sinking lungs dramatically secured the mother's acquittal.

After the Franco–Prussian war, Theophile Roussel (1816–1903) became an outstanding protagonist of the infant-welfare movement. The 'loi Roussel', of December 23, 1874, for the protection of infants sent out to nurse and his law of July 25, 1889, for the protection of abandoned and maltreated children earned him renown as 'the advocate of abandoned children', and led to a long continued social reform movement that extended well into the twentieth century (Garrison, 1965).

NATIONAL SOCIETY FOR THE PREVENTION OF CRUELTY TO CHILDREN

The first legal challenge to the absolute rights of parents over their children occurred in New York City in 1870 and it is interesting to observe that it took the persistence of an unnamed church worker and the society for the Prevention of Cruelty to Animals which had been founded 75 years earlier to instigate action. Fontana (1971) cites the interesting story of Mary Ellen, a small child living in New York City with her adoptive parents in 1871. The family was brought into court by a group of church workers due to severe abuse of the law, but no action was taken because child abuse was not against the law. Not to be outdone, the group had the parents brought into court with the assistance of the Society for the Prevention of Cruelty to Animals. Because Mary Ellen was technically a member of the animal kingdom, the case was heard and the child was removed from the parents. As a direct result of this incident many other societies with similar objectives were formed in different parts of the country. In Great Britain in 1899, 31 such societies united to form the National Society for the Prevention of Cruelty to Children (N.S.P.C.C.) with Queen Victoria as Patron and Parliament passed an act for prevention of cruelty to children which was dubbed 'The Children's Charter' (Allen and Morton, 1961).

Following the formation of the N.S.P.C.C. many other societies with similar objectives were formed. In New York City Samuel Halliday stirred public consciousness by working on behalf of destitute children (Radbill, 1968). In London Thomas Barnardo, forcing upon the public conscience awareness of the existence of gangs of homeless children, succeeded in the establishment of the chain of homes and vocational schools that earned for him the title 'Father of Nobody's Children' (Williams, 1966).

In conclusion it might be thought that maltreatment of children is an entity of the past. However, Fontana (1964) has asserted that child abuse is a disease of our times that 'has shown a steady increase in recent years'. An account of growing medical awareness and the steps taken by physicians and others in attempting to overcome a critical paediatric problem is, therefore, discussed in the next chapter.

Chapter 2

Modern Period of Medical Recognition

INTRODUCTION

Ambroise Tardieu, a French specialist in forensic medicine was the first to describe the medicosocial phenomenon of maltreated children in 1860. He also commented on child abuse in his work '*Étude Médico-Légale des Blessures*' (Medicolegal Study of Wounds) in 1860, quoted in Neimann and Rabouille (1969). In the first book on paediatrics ever written by an Englishman (and one of the earliest medical books printed in the English language), Thomas Phaire (1545), pointed to one of the social problems of his day – the phenomenon of neglect leading to hypothermia: 'Stifnes of limmes . . . which thyng procedeth many tymes of cold, as when a chylde is found in the frost, or in the strete, cast away by a wycked mother!'

The first case description in English of a battered child was read by Samuel West at a meeting of the Medical Society of London in 1888. He called his paper 'Acute Periosteal Swellings in Several Young Infants of the Same Family Probably Rickety in Nature'. From the summary of his cases below, West and his colleagues clearly misdiagnosed the condition;

> 'A child, aged 5 weeks, was brought by its mother, with the statement that its left arm had "dropped." A swelling occupied the middle third of the shaft of the humerus. Similar swellings were found on the right humerus and on the left femur. There were some slight bruises on the ribs. The patient was the fifth child. The first swelling came on the ninth day, the second in the fourth week, the last two days before it came under observation. Of the other children the eldest was similarly affected at the age of a week. The second was never so affected. The third and also the

> fourth were both affected. The second case was seen in a child of the brother of the father of the previous children. It was a girl infant aged three weeks and had developed a swelling of the left humerus a week before being seen. This patient was the fourth child. The first had always been well. The second had both arms and legs affected in the same way at the same age. That these were cases of early rickets could not, however, be doubted, on account of the evidence of rickets in the family and the absence of any other assignable cause.'
>
> (West, 1888)

In the discussion that followed this paper (West, 1888), several physicians indicated their doubts that rickets was responsible for this strange disease. The multiplicity of the lesions, the fact that 'the stress of the disease fell on the middle shaft', and that the symptoms appeared very early, even among infants who were breast fed, were cited as arguments against a diagnosis of rickets. It is interesting to note that none of the physicians present at that meeting suggested that maltreatment by the parents might be an alternative explanation.

These early reports of battered children antedated the discovery of the x-ray in 1895 and were not, therefore, substantiated. Although great advances were made in most areas of x-ray diagnosis immediately following the introduction of x-rays, the radiographic features of injuries to bones of infants and their repair were not described in detail until almost 40 years later when Snedecor, Knapp and Wilson (1935) described the bizarre radiographic manifestations of recovery from epiphyseal separation during breech extraction. At about the same time articles on unusual periosteal reactions in children which were primarily to be differentiated from those of congenital syphilis began to make their appearance (Rose, 1936; Caffey, 1939).

The concept of the 'battered child' and the recent developments in the elucidation of the condition are intimately related to the field of diagnostic radiology. Historically the initial recognition of this syndrome was primarily by virtue of radiological studies. It is fascinating to examine this early radiological literature for it shows how interest was stimulated by papers published primarily in radiological journals.

EARLY RADIOLOGICAL REPORTS OF BATTERED CHILDREN

The modern period of medical recognition began in the middle 1940s with the appearance of several articles by Caffey and his associates on a 'new syndrome' (Caffey and Silverman, 1945): 'For many years we have been puzzled by the roentgen disclosures of fresh, healing and healed multiple fractures in the long bones of infants whose principal disease was chronic subdural hematoma' (Caffey, 1946*a*). In another paper published in the same year (Caffey, 1946*b*) he wrote:

> 'During the Spring of 1938 we studied an infant whose principle lesions were scattered swellings deep in the soft tissues and scattered cortical thickenings in several bones. After extensive investigation it is evident that this patient suffered from none of the recognized conditions in which cortical thickenings have been found previously, such as scurvy, rickets, syphilis, bacterial osteitis, neoplastic disease, or traumatic injury. The three findings common to all of our patients were: (*1*) tender swelling deep in the soft tissues; (*2*) cortical thickening in the skeleton; and (*3*) onset during the first three months of life. Other manifestations which were present in some patients but lacking in others were fever, pleurisy, anaemia and increase in the sedimentation rate of the erythrocytes . . . after prolonged investigation of four patients, the cause remained undetermined . . . Traumatic injury was not observed in a single case either at home or in hospital'.

Caffey raised many questions in this article. What is the nature of this strange disease? Why was there blood in the vomit and faeces? Why were there bluish and black spots on the face and arms? Why were there fresh fractures, some in the process of healing and some already healed? Why were some of the children pale and undernourished? Why do they get better in hospital and worse after discharge? Caffey (1946*a*) cites an example of this last question by referring to one infant who was discharged after a month in hospital:

> 'Four days later the mother brought the baby back to hospital because the right leg had suddenly become tender and swollen and bruises had appeared under the left eye and in other parts of the body. The mother denied that any injury had occurred during the four days since discharge from hospital. Roentgenograms of the extremities disclosed that the bones in the arms were normal, but five fractures were visible in the shafts of the bones adjacent to the knee joints. The patient remained in hospital for twenty-five days. The swellings and tenderness gradually disappeared'.

Caffey considered a number of possible explanations for the phenomena he observed; that children injured themselves during convulsions, that skeletal disease so weakened the bones that they were unusually vulnerable to trauma or that the children were suffering from scurvy. He rejected all these explanations and suggested instead that 'recognized injuries may be denied by mothers or nurses because injury to an infant implies negligence on the part of its caretaker' (Caffey, 1946*a*). Accepting the views of Ingraham and Heyl (1939), that the subdural haematomas were traumatic, Caffey (1946*a*) suggested a traumatic origin for these injuries also – 'Some of the fractures in the long bones were caused by the same traumatic forces which presumably were responsible for the subdural hematoma'.

Ample support for Caffey's observations of bone lesions with subdural haematoma quickly followed (Lis and Frauenberger, 1950; Smith, 1950; Marquézy, Bach and Blondeau, 1952; Bakwin, 1952).

In 1953, Silverman, following Caffey's lead, insisted on a traumatic basis for injuries of the type now known to occur in the battered child in a presentation of three cases of the condition without subdural haematomas:

> 'It is not often appreciated that many individuals responsible for the care of infants and children . . . may permit trauma and be unaware of it, may recognize trauma but forget or be reluctant to admit it, or may deliberately injure the child and deny it.'
>
> (Silverman, 1953)

Astley (1953) suggested that the aetiology was a primary metaphyseal fragility of bone in affected children, but this concept was discarded by Woolley and Evans in 1955. These authors reviewed material seen over a period of 8 years with radiographic findings suggesting injury, with or without a history of trauma. They concluded that the radiographic manifestations of injury and its repair were identical whether a history of injury was or was not obtained and that the skeletal lesions 'having the appearance of fracture, regardless of history of injury or presence or absence of intracranial bleeding – are due to undesirable vectors of force' (Woolley and Evans, 1955). They also emphasized that the environmental factors surrounding such infants frequently included grossly undesirable and hazardous circumstances. Subsequent papers have since appeared which reinforced and confirmed Woolley and Evans' conclusions (Bakwin, 1956; Jones and Davis, 1957; Weston, 1957; Fisher, 1958; Friedman, 1958; Miller, 1959; Altman and Smith, 1960; Gwinn, Lewin and Peterson, (1961).

In 1956 at the Mackenzie Davidson Memorial Lecture in London, Caffey spoke of the importance of early diagnosis in saving abused children from further injury and dealt in detail with the radiological aspects:

> 'The correct early diagnosis of injury may be the only means by which abused youngsters can be removed from their traumatic environment and their wrongdoers punished. Correct early diagnosis of injury may be life-saving to some of these otherwise helpless youngsters, or it may prevent permanent crippling injuries to others.'
>
> (Caffey, 1957)

In discussing how the truth is avoided by physicians, Caffey indicated that the radiologist had 'to stand his ground . . . and urge his trauma-insensitive colleagues to go into the history of trauma more fully, and when necessary make a searching investigation himself' (Caffey, 1957). The latter advice was in marked contrast to the generally accepted obligation of physicians in such cases.

The evidence of the radiological signs of bone injury and repair provided the medical foundation upon which was built the social, legal and psychiatric aspects of the problem.

THE BATTERED CHILD SYNDROME

C. Henry Kempe, a paediatrician at the University of Colorado School of Medicine was alarmed, in the early sixties, by the large number of children admitted under his care who were suffering from non-accidental injury. In order to obtain a more accurate picture of the true incidence of the problem he and his colleagues (Kempe *et al.*, 1962) undertook a nationwide survey of hospitals and reported their findings as follows:

> 'Among 71 hospitals replying 302 cases were reported to have occurred in a one-year period; 33 of the children died and 85 suffered permanent brain injury. In one-third of the cases proper medical diagnosis was followed by some type of legal action. We also surveyed 77 District Attorney's who reported that they had knowledge of 447 cases in a similar one-year period. Of these 45 died and 29 suffered permanent brain damage; court action was initiated in 46 per cent of this group.'

To direct attention to the seriousness of the problem these authors proposed the term 'battered child syndrome' which they defined in the following way:

> 'A term used by us to characterize a clinical condition in young children who have received serious physical abuse, generally from a parent or foster parent. The syndrome should be considered in any child exhibiting evidence of fracture of any bone, subdural hematoma, failure to thrive, soft tissue swelling or skin bruising, in any child who dies suddenly, or where the degree and type of injury is at variance with the history given regarding the occurrence of the trauma.'

Kempe *et al.* (1962) also pointed out that psychiatric factors were probably of prime importance in the pathogenesis of the disorder, but that knowledge of such factors was limited. They concluded that physical abuse was a major cause of death and maiming among children, and discussed the reluctance of physicians to accept the possibility of parental abuse and to take an investigative role. Because of this they recommended that physicians report all incidents to law enforcement authorities or child protective agencies.

An editorial in the *Journal of the American Medical Association* (1962), commented favourably on this article and recommended that doctors be alert to battered baby cases and co-operate with law enforcement agencies.

ALTERNATIVE TERMINOLOGY

The term 'battered child syndrome' (Kempe *et al.*, 1962) or 'battered baby syndrome' (British Paediatric Association, 1966) is so emotive (Cooper, 1970) that perhaps it should be dropped. Caffey (1972) suggests that the chief drawback is that it tends to provoke and inflame the hearer, and spark a premature bias against accused parents before adequate medical and legal investigations can be made. Instead he has proposed the term 'Parent–Infant Traumatic Stress Syndrome', which is a fair name, accuses no one and 'does indicate the casual, emotional, social and economic stresses which plague the mother or her substitute'. By way of contrast Cameron (1971), favours 'Battered Baby' on the grounds that it describes the situation very clearly and is useful diagnostically.

Other innocuous terms have also been suggested: 'Multiple Epiphyseal Injuries' (Griffiths and Moynihan, 1963); 'Caffey's Third Syndrome', (Fairburn and Hunt, 1964); 'The Syndrome of Ambroise Tardieu' (Silverman, 1972); 'Silverman's Syndrome' (Maroteaux and Fessard, 1969); 'Caffey–Kempe Syndrome' (Caffey, 1972); 'Unrecognized Trauma' (Silverman, 1972); 'Unsuspected Trauma in Infancy' (Gwinn, Lewin and Peterson, 1961); 'Traumatic Periostitis' (Barmeyer, Alderson and Cox, 1951). Other terms mentioned in the literature include: 'Traumatization of Children' (Snedeker, 1962); 'Ill-Treated Child Syndrome' (Cameron, 1970); 'Parental Dysfunction' (Galdston, 1965); 'Physical Ill-Treatment of Children' (Isaacs, 1968) and 'The Maltreated Child' (Fontana, 1971).

Due to the difficulty of pigeon-holing all cases, Camps, (quoted in Cameron, 1971), has suggested four main subdivisions of the battered child syndrome each overlapping in aetiology.

Type 1 – True Infanticide

In these cases the mother kills the child within a short time of birth using various methods easily at hand; smothering, drowning, cutting, strangling or bashing. In many instances there is little firm evidence that childbirth or lactation has anything to do with the killing. However, psychiatric factors precipitated by similar conditions as occurring in Type 4 play a part.

Type 2 – The Wasted and Neglected Child

Such children are grossly underweight and ill-fed even though adequate food is available. They also show evidence of napkin rash and other septic lesions. Their mothers are unusually inadequate and their homes are also neglected.

Type 3 – Deliberate Cruelty

These children are beaten with a stick or belt, burnt with cigarette ends or hot objects, scalded, deliberately deprived of fluids and shut in cupboards. They may also be wasted from malnutrition. A particular child is usually singled out by a cruel and rejecting parent.

Type 4 – The Battered Child

These children are adequately cared for in terms of food, clothing and toys. However, in most cases there is evidence of repetitive injuries and in many medical aid has been sought on several occasions for fractures of the long bones or other injuries. One third of these children are illegitimate, pre-maritally conceived or unwanted by their young and low-intelligence parents.

Fontana (1971) has similarly argued that baby battering is at one end of a spectrum and has proposed the term 'Maltreatment Syndrome in Children'.

> 'A more precise and descriptive term that should be applied to this clinical entity is the 'maltreatment syndrome in children.' A maltreated child often presents itself without obvious signs of being battered but with the multiple minor physical evidences of emotional and, at times, nutritional deprivation, neglect and abuse. The battered child is only the last phase of the spectrum of the maltreatment syndrome.'

'The Maltreatment Syndrome' is also the preferred term of some Australian (Birrell and Birrell, 1968), and French authors (Tabibian, 1969; Neimann and Rabouille, 1969). 'Kindesmisshandlung', is the equivalent term used in Germany (Köttgen, 1967). The degree of overlap between each of the categories and the evidence that baby battering is at one end of a spectrum, as Camps and Fontana suggest, will be discussed later.

Though 'Child Abuse' is the heading listed in the *Cummulative Medical Index,* other terminology frequently appears in the literature. These include: 'Violent Cruelty to Children' (Gibbens and Walker, 1956); 'Cruelty to Children' (Fleming, 1967); 'Child Abuse Syndrome' (Silver, Dublin and Lourie, 1969*a*); 'The Abused Child Complex' (Krige, 1966); 'The Physically Abused Child' (Bain, 1963); 'Physical Abuse of Children' (Merrill, 1962; Gill, 1969) and 'Ill-Treated Children' (Oliver and Taylor, 1971).

Gibson (1973) has suggested that some of these terms are euphemistic expressions that maintain public complacency. He prefers the term 'Grievous Bodily Harm', on the grounds that it expresses accurately 'the nature of the injuries in cases of assault and battery upon any individual' and would 'also ensure that no one section of the community by privilege or intellect or position, could continually investigate, diagnose and treat both parties'. Mounsey (1975) has pointed out that the definition of these cases rests with the police.

> 'Non-Accidental Injuries to children are usually crimes classified by the law of this land under one of the following headings: Murder, Attempted Murder, Manslaughter, Infanticide, Child Destruction, Wounding, Assaults, Cruelty to Children and Young Persons'.

Kempe (1973) has aptly described the difficulty of terminology:

> 'The definition of child abuse and neglect is not what the doctor thinks it should be, or what the social worker thinks it is, but is actually what the court says it is. The court is, of course, influenced by the public, and its definition will change from time to time and may be different in differing localities, based on the emotional climate of the cities in that area'.

The operational definition used in our 1973 study (Smith, Hanson and Noble, 1973) was 'Inadequately or Unexplained Injuries'. This was not to complicate the issue further but it was felt that it best described the clinical picture in a non-emotional fashion and accounted for the majority of cases seen in hospital practice. 'Non-Accidental Injury' is another term that has recently evolved from the workings of the Tunbridge Wells Study Group (1973). Neither of these terms has yet supplanted the diagnostic label of 'Battered Child Syndrome' (W.H.O., 1968) and throughout this book, therefore, some of these terms will be used interchangeably.

BABY BATTERING: A GLOBAL PHENOMENON

A large number of reports were also published from many other countries during the 1960s. In the U.S.A. Fontana, Donovan and Wong

(1963); Fontana (1964, 1966, 1968); Luke, Lyons and Devlin (1967); Silver, Dublin and Lourie (1969*a*, *b*) and many other authors published papers on the battered child syndrome. In France, under the impetus of articles by Professor Neimann of the Nancy School of Paediatrics, French medical opinion was also aroused. The 'idiopathic' nature of subdural haematomata was demystified when he showed that such trauma was a result of parental cruelty (Neimann and Rabouille, 1969). Gormsen and Vesterdal in Denmark also provided detailed accounts of the injuries these children experienced. In their series, which was collected mainly from the Forensic Institute of Copenhagen, the mortality rate was 55 per cent (Vesterdal, 1972).

In Sweden a Government Committee (Chairman: Professor R. Zetterström) reported a series of 119 maltreated children belonging to 106 families. Fifteen of these children were killed and 44 were severely injured. Most of the children were under 3 years of age. Twenty-two children had one or more fractures. Some of the survivors showed signs of psychological disturbances, such as depression and pseudoretardation. Twenty-four children had previously been admitted to hospitals on account of lesions which might have been caused by maltreatment but were not diagnosed as such (quoted in Vesterdal, 1972).

Tabibibian (1969) described nine cases he had examined at the Geneva University Children's Hospital and emphasized the importance of psychological assessment. Numerous other cases were also reported from England, Switzerland, France, Belgium and Germany during the 1960s (Vesterdal, 1972). In Australia, Storey alerted doctors by reporting six cases he had seen while working overseas: 'The case histories are presented to emphasize the presence of this entity and to stimulate members of the medical profession to be aware of the condition' (Storey, 1964). Birrell and Birrell (1968) reported a series of 42 maltreated children seen at the Royal Children's Hospital in Melbourne. They discussed the clinical and radiological features of the syndrome and emphasized that repetitive injury was common. In suggesting a programme to improve management they pleaded for 'power to remove children at grave risk' from their abusive environments. The complacency which existed north of the Victorian border is evident from the following statement which appeared in a Sydney evening newspaper several months before Birrell and Birrell's report was published.

> 'All I can say is that New South Wales does not have a battered baby problem, maybe it's the difference in climate but there's certainly no problem in this state'.
>
> (*Daily Mirror*, 21st March, 1968)

Callaghan and Fotheringham (1970), however, emphasized the wide ranging degree of psychopathology among baby batterers and outlined initial treatment and interview techniques to the Australian medical profession.

In New Zealand, Gluckman (1968) suggested a psychiatric classification of parents who maltreated children and discussed the difficulties confronting doctors when dealing with a case. In Canada, the clinical, legal and moral problems were discussed by Pashayan and Cochrane (1965) and Maxwell (1966); Blue (1965), outlined the social aspects of the phenomenon. Several British authors published articles in foreign medical journals; Simpson (1968) outlined the characteristic clinical features of battered children to the South African Medical profession and Bennie and Sclare (1969) reported the psychopathology of 10 baby batterers to American doctors.

Bwibo (1971) has described a case of a Ugandan boy aged 8 years who presented with swelling of the face, eyelids and hands. The preliminary diagnosis was acute glomerulonephritis. It was only after negative tests and repeated questioning that the child admitted being beaten by his uncle. Paul (1972) has suggested that 'in India there is a need for the formation of legislation for the protection of the battered child', and has advised his Indian colleagues 'not . . . to return the child to an environment where even a moderate risk of repetition exists'.

The Battered Child Syndrome is thus seen to have no geographical boundaries. The 'Child Abuse' heading appeared for the first time in the *Cummulative Index Medicus* in 1965 and gave 32 references. Since then there has been an average annual listing of 40 references from most countries on the globe.

GROWING AWARENESS IN BRITAIN

Attention was aroused in Britain with the publication of Griffiths and Moynihan's case reports in 1963. These emphasized the importance of multiple epiphyseal injuries. Publications confirming other cases quickly followed (Fairburn and Hunt, 1964; Simpson, 1965, 1967; Cameron, Johnson and Camps, 1966). In 1966 a memorandum 'The Battered Baby' prepared by the Special Standing Committee on Accidents in Childhood (British Paediatric Association) was published. This memorandum made comprehensive recommendations to doctors concerning the action to be taken when there was suspicion of willful injury to a child and quoted extracts from statutes thought relevant to dealing with such cases. This advice on management was reiterated by Fleming in 1967. The Medical Defence Union (1966) also issued a statement in its Annual Report concerning the management of battered babies.

In 1969 the National Society for the Prevention of Cruelty to Children established a 'Battered Child Research Department' which shortly after its formation published a report; '78 battered children: a retrospective study' (Skinner and Castle, 1969). This study resulted from an analysis of the case records of 78 battered children who came to the notice of the N.S.P.C.C. in 1 year, from 1st July, 1967 to 30th June, 1968, and who had been physically injured to an extent serious enough to warrant medical attention. The findings from this report are summarized below.

In the sample of battered children (all of whom were under 4 years of age), 56 per cent were less than 1 year old and the modal age was 2 months. All except seven of the children had been admitted to hospital on account of their injuries. Two out of every five who were discharged home after hospital treatment had to be re-admitted on account of a subsequent injury. The authors commented that such unsatisfactory aftercare arrangements made by hospitals, despite evidence of repeated unexplained injury are disturbing. The study showed that bruises and injuries which appeared to be of minor nature, could signify the beginning of increasing violent forms of injury to the child. The high incidence of trauma to the face (43.5 per cent) may, like bruising, be an aid to early diagnosis of a nurturing problem, which if modified could avert serious injury to a child.

The findings also questioned the assumption that radiological evidence was essential to the diagnosis of a battered child, and indicated that to wait for such evidence before protecting the child could have serious consequences. The study showed that in families where the first child was battered there was a 13:1 chance that a subsequent child would be injured; a finding of particular importance to all those who had to weigh the risks of supervised home care for the battered child against an alternative protective course of action. Although the sample was small the study showed that the prematurity incidence was twice the national average.

The battering adults were in most cases between 20 and 30 years of age, married and with a small family. Women were responsible for battering in just over half the incidents, but there was evidence of collusion by their partners in many cases. They appeared to have longstanding emotional problems which were highlighted by the demands and responsibilities of parenthood. Though not verified with the criminal records office Skinner and Castle reported that at least 45 per cent of the men were known to have criminal records, mostly for larceny and crimes of violence. They were also unemployed at the time of the incident. Many of the battering females were either pregnant or recently confined. The families tended to move from their accommodation at crises times, and were socially isolated.

RECOMMENDATIONS FROM THE DEPARTMENT OF HEALTH AND SOCIAL SECURITY

In February, 1970, the Chief Medical Officer of the Home Office Children's Department wrote jointly to Medical Officers of Health of Local Health Authorities and to Children's Officers asking them to consult together on the problem of the 'battered child' in their area and to bring others involved into their discussions (Central Health Service Council, 1970). It was suggested that representatives of the local Medical Committee, paediatricians, consultants responsible for accident departments, the police and social agencies such as the N.S.P.C.C. should review together the situation in their own area and decide what further arrangements could be made to ensure that all necessary protection and assistance could be made available to the child, to others at risk in the family and to the parents and other adults. Moreover it was recommended that such a group could have a continuing function in reviewing the local situation from time to time.

Medical Officers of Health and Children's Officers were asked to prepare progress reports on their consultations. Later in the year while these reports were being compiled, the Department of Health and Social Security issued a memorandum which was prepared by the Standing Medical Advisory Committee (Central Health Services Council, 1970) and which dealt in general terms with both the individual and general management aspects of the syndrome.

In May 1972 the Department of Health and Social Security published an analysis of the reports asked for (D.H.S.S., 1972). The reports received indicated certain common problems. The organization and management patterns of local authorities closely reflected the advice given in the memorandum, which pointed out that, although firm diagnosis is rarely possible at the earliest stage, a suspicion of the syndrome may be aroused in the minds of any of those who make the first professional contact with the child. The memorandum considered the parts which the health visitor, general practitioner, the hospital accident and emergency staff, and the social worker all might play individually and collectively, and concluded that a team approach is essential if protection is to be given to the child and aid to the family.

The reports of Medical Officers of Health and Children's Officers made it clear that the concentration of thinking and resources were in the diagnosis, immediate treatment and prevention of repetition of child abuse. The reports also pointed out the importance of research, prevention and long-term treatment for the families once the crisis period was over but contained little specific information on these aspects. The analysis of the reports submitted stressed that there were four key issues of the problem; prevention of child abuse, social and medical action when it is suspected, action on diagnosis, and subsequent rehabilitation of the families concerned and discussed each of these aspects in turn. It was suggested that the establishment of a two-tiered system of case conferences for individual families, and of area review committees to oversee the general feasibility of plans would improve management.

> 'The theme running through all the reports received is that all local authorities are doing their best in the face of a very difficult problem and are diligently seeking ways to improve the management of the problem in their own area.'
>
> (D.H.S.S., 1972)

RECENT DEVELOPMENTS

The management and treatment of battered children present in the first instance clinical problems for which the doctor must, of course, assume clinical responsibility. His primary aim is to treat the injury and protect the child from further harm; his ultimate aim is to rehabilitate the family. Because these aims cannot be achieved alone and because of an increasing number and continuing series of deaths (4000–5000 battered children per year in Britain with a 10 per cent mortality rate), the Tunbridge Wells Study Group was established in May 1973 and shortly after published a report and resolutions. The author was invited to join the study group (Chairman: Dr. Alfred White Franklin) and others present represented most of the professional bodies concerned with the problem. The papers presented by each member at this meeting have recently been compiled as a book (White Franklin, 1975).

The Study Group supported the suggestion of the Department of Health and Social Security (1972) recommending a two-tiered system of management; case conferences about individual families and area review committees to oversee the general feasibility of plans. However, the Group proposed a clearer description of function of this system and some modifications in composition. The Department of Health and Social Security gave the widest possible circulation to the Report and Resolutions and the British Paediatric Association and British Association of Paediatric Surgeons commented favourably on its recommendations (Nixon and Court, 1973). The two associations, through a special committee, are keeping the whole subject under continuing review, and are currently seeking their members' comments on the study group's resolutions.

Over the past few years several working groups have been established in various regions throughout Britain. Under the Chairmanship of the late Dr. Carey Smallwood, Birmingham was one of the first regions in Britain that disseminated information to interested agencies and encouraged doctors to use a 'Request for Information Card'. This working party has recently been replaced by the 'Birmingham Area Review Committee on Non-Accidental Injury'. Its members comprise those detailed in the Tunbridge Wells Study Group report. A similar working party in Newcastle (Chairman: Professor John Webb) have recently published '*A Guide on Management*' (*Non-Accidental Injury in Children, 1973*) which represents a local code of professional practice but which should also be of value to other centres.

More recently, the Chief Medical Officer, Chief Nursing Officer and Director of the Social Work Services, have widely circulated a document that has underlined the need for regular joint review of all aspects of the management of cases and has requested that area review committees be established for this purpose (D.H.S.S., 1974). The Secretary of State has also requested a report at the end of 1974 from these committees.

It is, of course, too early to assess the results of these recent developments in reducing the prevalence of baby battering. The recommendations from all the above groups, once established, should however go a long way towards improving management and developing the essential cooperation between all the professional workers involved.

Chapter 3

Clinical Manifestations of the Battered Child Syndrome

INTRODUCTION

Literature on the medical aspects of child abuse is extensive. The edited volumes of Helfer and Kempe (1968); Kempe and Helfer (1972) and Fontana's (1971) monograph, provides a general overview as do the articles by Paulson and Blake (1967); Silver (1968) and Zalba (1966). A thorough bibliography on child abuse was published by the United States Department of Health, Education and Welfare (1969). The National Library of Medicine (1973) has also published a literature search produced by the Library's Medical Literature Analyses and Retrieval System (MEDLARS) which lists 303 articles on the battered child syndrome. A selected list of references has also been recently published by the Department of Health and Social Security Library (1973). The following section reviews the literature that describes the common clinical manifestations of the battered child syndrome.

MEDICAL ASPECTS

SURFACE MARKS

These consist of bruises, abrasions and burns of different colours and clearly of different ages, indicative of repeated incidents (Cameron, 1970). Though children bruise easily, the important factor in diagnosis is the distribution of the bruises (Cameron, 1970). Cameron, Johnson and Camps (1966) consider that laceration of the mucosa of the lip from the alveolar margin of the gum is pathognomonic. This injury which was present in 50 per cent of their series is thought to result from a blow on the mouth or other efforts to silence a screaming or crying child. A clue to diagnosis is also provided by the presence of a subgaleal haematoma. 'The most likely cause of childhood subgaleal hematoma is a vigorous hair-pull by the grip of an enraged adult' (Hamlin, 1968).

Sussman (1968), has described four characteristics which distinguish skin lesions in the battered child syndrome from other skin lesions.

(1) The lesions are often concentrated in clusters on the trunk and buttocks and, to a lesser extent, on the head and proximal segments of extremities.
(2) The lesions are morphologically similar to the implements used to inflict trauma. The hand, belt buckle, strap, rope, burning cigarette or match or other instruments have been identified as weapons used to traumatize a child and they produce bleeding and characteristic straight, curvilinear, circular or jagged lesions.
(3) Bleeding into the skin is purpuric – and almost never petechial – and it is distributed among the abrasions and scratches.
(4) The skin lesions are of different ages and, in this respect, bear some similarity to the bony pathology.

In distinguishing these skin lesions from those incurred in an accident or during play, Sussman (1968) observed that the latter are usually of similar age, have non-specific and ill-defined shapes, and are commonly found on the extremities.

The limbs frequently show 'finger-tip' bruises commonly grouped around the elbows and knees, due to gripping the child so as to shake or pull him or hurl him into his cot or against furniture, while more diffuse bruises may be due to blows or impact against a surface. Bruising of the chest and trunk may be due to blows, while bruising to the abdominal wall is often minimal, in spite of severe intra-abdominal injury. It is often difficult, due to shock and peripheral vascular failure, to age the bruises with accuracy. 'The degree of trauma provided in the histories frequently cannot explain the severity of the injuries' (Cameron, 1970).

VISCERAL INJURIES

Additional acute problems requiring immediate surgical consultation have been reported. Gastric or intestinal perforations and intestinal obstruction have been seen as a result of trauma (Eisenstein, Delta and Clifford, 1965; McCort and Vaudagna, 1964; Kempe, 1971).

Liver, spleen and kidney lacerations, as well as haematomas in the lumen of the small bowel causing acute obstruction are also reasonably common. Pseudocyst of the pancreas, a rare condition in childhood, has also been described (Bongiovi and Logosso, 1969) as a result of baby battering.

Cameron (1970) has pointed out that rupture of the liver and abdominal viscera with tearing of the mesentery is common. A decelerating force, such as a punch or blow, tears the mesentery and may disrupt the small intestine at sites of ligamental support. Such a blow to a relaxed abdomen may cause severe intestinal injury and yet leave no external mark.

Other studies have also described the varieties of visceral injuries that may occur. Camps (1969) reported 19 liver injuries in 100 fatal cases of battered children. Touloukian (1968) reported one liver injury in five necropsy studies and McCort and Vaudagna (1964) reported another two cases of liver injury and one of them was fatal. Simpson (1965) reported a conviction for murder after the death of siblings, both of whom suffered liver rupture.

Gornall *et al.* (1972) reported six battered children suffering from intra-abdominal visceral injuries who were treated in the children's hospitals of Manchester. They showed that epigastric and small intestinal injuries predominated and in this respect the pattern of trauma differed from that seen in children injured in road traffic and other accidents. Delay in referral contributed strongly to the death of two of the battered children.

OPHTHALMIC MANIFESTATIONS

Ocular damage, though not a common manifestation, has also been described. A review of the rather sparse literature available on this subject shows that the principal manifestations of the battered baby syndrome which have been described previously are; injuries to the eyelids (Woolley and Evans, 1955; Cameron, Johnson and Camps, 1966), posterior subcapsular cataracts (Kiffney, 1964), peripheral choroidoretinal atrophy (Maroteaux and Lamy, 1967) and pre-retinal and retinal haemorrhages (Gilkes and Mann, 1967). Mushin (1971) and Harcourt and Hopkins (1971), in describing a series of battered baby cases with ocular damage, stressed the frequency of permanent visual impairment that occurs in this condition, and underlined the necessity for a complete ophthalmic examination in all such cases.

NEUROLOGICAL ASPECTS

Several authors (Kempe *et al.*, 1962; Baron, Bejar and Sheaff, 1970; Silber and Bell, 1971; Guthkelch, 1971) have described the neurological sequelae that may result from battering. Subdural haematoma is common (Guthkelch, 1971) and occurred in 42 per cent of Weston's series (1968). Kempe *et al.* (1962) noted that in their experience the extremeties of the child are often used as handles during an episode of rough treatment; 'sometimes an arm is pulled to jerk a reluctant child to his feet, sometimes the legs are held when a tiny baby is swung in a punitive way'. In one of Caffey's (1946*a*) cases of subdural haematoma the history is given in the following words. 'Baby rolled off a table and his mother grabbed him by the forearm and jerked him in the air to prevent his fall.' Guthkelch (1971) has described how children with subdural haematoma may have no external marks of injury on the head and suggested that repeated acceleration or deceleration (whiplash injury) rather than direct violence is the cause of the haemorrhage. In Weston's (1968) series of fatal cases there were three children who had subdural haematoma but no external bruising to the head; the assailants admitted they had shaken their child violently. Court (1969), quoted a mother's confession that she was in the habit of shaking her babies 'in an insane rage'. Direct trauma has also been described and is possibly a more common cause of intracranial bleeding. Lukianowicz (1971) mentioned one father who used 'to hammer the child with his fist, mostly hitting him on the head'. A variety of other different instruments have also been described as being used by battering parents (Helfer and Kempe, 1968).

In the series of Kempe *et al.* (1962) 15 per cent of the survivors were left with cerebral palsy. Growth failure and developmental retardation have also been described as occurring frequently (Gregg, 1968; Fontana, Donovan and Wong, 1963; Elmer and Gregg, 1967; Patton and Gardner, 1962; Martin, 1972). Baron, Bejar and Sheaff (1970) have suggested that the battered child syndrome 'be included in the differential diagnosis of developmental failure with diffuse nonfocal neurologic signs and all infants who show these symptoms should be hospitalized'. Silber and Bell (1971) have emphasized the importance of having a high index of suspicion when confronted by such cases and have described six battered babies with craniocerebral trauma that caused diagnostic confusion. The most serious error that is made in the evaluation of children with possible head injury is the absence of frequent serial head measurements (Helfer and Pollock, 1968). Several cases of spine and spinal cord trauma have been described (Swischuk,

1969) and Fiser, Kaplan and Holder (1972) have detailed how a battered child can mimic the pseudoparalysis of congenital syphilis.

Although there have been no long-term prospective studies on the consequences and sequelae of child abuse, Martin's (1972) short-term follow-up study has shown that permanent damage to the brain is a frequent sequela of physical abuse. Forty-three per cent of his series showed neurological abnormalities at follow-up examination. Sixty-six per cent of these children had obvious neurological impairment; hemiparesis, focal signs, optic atrophy and pathological primitive reflexes. The other 33.3 per cent had more subtle signs, which included various 'soft' neurological findings with minimal brain dysfunction. Of these 18 children with neurological dysfunction, only 50 per cent had a history of skull fracture or subdural haematoma, which suggested that brain damage was related to less dramatic trauma. Although nearly 50 per cent of the brain-damaged children had normal intelligence, Martin (1972), suggested that their handicaps would preclude success at school.

Morse, Sahler and Friedman (1970) followed up 25 children for approximately 3 years after hospitalization for battering. During this follow-up period, 33.3 per cent of the children had again been battered or neglected. Assessing their intellectual, emotional and social development the authors judged 70 per cent of the children to be outside the normal range. In evaluating the types and effectiveness of intervention by community agencies the study disclosed that more attention to rehabilitating these families is vitally needed.

THERMAL AND CAUSTIC MANIFESTATIONS

'Intentional burning of children as a form of child abuse is probably more common than heretofore suspected' (Stone *et al.*, 1970). However, there have been only isolated reports of child abuse by burning. Gillespie (1965) described 19 patients with thermal and caustic manifestations; the manner of infliction of the burns he described reflect the tormenting capacity of the parents. Scalding liquids, usually water and coffee, accounted for the burns in 11 instances. Six patients had scalding water thrown upon them and one infant was fed boiling milk. Two children had caustic burns of the mouth and pharynx. This occurred when they were forced to rinse their mouths with drain cleanser because they had eaten their parents' dessert. The perineum was the most frequent site of burns. Three children were placed in contact with a hot stove and one patient was thrown on the heating grate of a floor surface. Burns by contact with cigarettes occurred in one child and cremation was attempted in one infant. Apart from actual burns, frostbite was encountered in two patients. This injury occurred when the children were forced to take a bath in slush and snow and remain out of doors as punishment for a minor disobedience. The frostbite in each instance was complicated by pneumonia and malnutrition. Gillespie (1965), who reported his findings at the Twenty Fourth Annual Session of the Association for the Surgery of Trauma, advised his colleagues as follows:

> 'Thermal and caustic injuries occur in the syndrome with a greater frequency than had been previously identified . . . unless the true nature of these injuries is recognized, a repetitious pattern develops leading to permanent disability and occasionally death.'

A similar conclusion was reached by Stone *et al.* (1970) at Cook County Hospital in Chicago. These authors found that burns were the primary injury in over 10 per cent of child abuse cases and were a secondary diagnosis in an additional 7 per cent. Five (19 per cent) of the victims died as a result of the burns. They also advised that 'the physicians treating the burn-abused child can obviously not prevent the first episode of abuse, but he must accept responsibility for attempting to preclude subsequent episodes'.

RADIOLOGICAL ASPECTS

Silverman (1968) has reviewed the radiological aspects at length and shown that films taken too early after the initial trauma may fail to detect changes in the long bones. It is the healing process that is seen in many cases rather than the acute trauma or fracture, and for this reason he has suggested that x-rays should be repeated in 2–3 weeks if the original films are negative. 'To the informed clinician, the bones tell a story the child is too young or too frightened to tell' (Cameron, 1970).

The outstanding features of skeletal injuries in the battered child syndrome have also been described in detail by Caffey (1946*a*). Gwinn, Lewin and Peterson (1961) have reported a series of 25 cases of unsuspected trauma in a period of 2 years. Krige (1966) pointed out that the predominant findings are radiological and that doctors are often astounded by the severity and extent of the pathology revealed.

Predilection for epiphyses, exaggerated periosteal reaction, multiplicity of lesions and differing stages of healing and repair of the multiple lesions are characteristic of this condition. Repeated pulling and twisting of an infants' long bones result in epiphyseal separation and subperiosteal haemorrhage in the metaphyseal and epiphyseal areas.

This haemorrhage is followed by a healing process resulting in callus formation which is quite diagnostic (Silverman, 1968). The presence of such findings on x-ray, associated with other evidence of recurrent trauma, confirms the diagnosis of the battered child syndrome. Caffey (1965), however, has rightfully expressed caution and insists that a great deal of care be used in making this diagnosis.

Although radiological changes are rarely confused with many other conditions, Silverman (1968) has listed several entities that should be considered in the differential diagnosis. These include: epiphyseal separation from known trauma, scurvy, syphilis, osteogenesis imperfecta, infantile cortical hyperostosis, osteid oesteoma, fatigue fractures, 'little league elbow', neurogenic sensory deficit and congenital indifference to pain. The Ehlers–Danlos syndrome has also been reported to cause some confusion in diagnosis (Barabas, 1967). In paediatric practice, however, it is most unusual to confuse any of the above diagnoses with the battered child syndrome (Helfer and Pollock, 1968). The diagnosis may not be recognized, however, because 'many physicians find it hard to believe that such an attack could have occurred and they attempt to obliterate such suspicions from their mind even in the face of obvious circumstantial evidence' (Kempe *et al.*, 1962).

OTHER CLINICAL MANIFESTATIONS

A variety of other clinical manifestations have been described. Manson (1964) was the first to describe the association of the coeliac syndrome (malabsorption) and parental abuse. In one of his three cases the patient had not only been starved but showed other clinical features characteristic of baby battering. Kunstadter, Singer and Steinberg (1967) also described a case of coeliac syndrome induced by starvation and reported 'that physical abuse, neglect and/or emotional trauma may be responsible for the celiac syndrome' Kunstadter, Singer and Steinberg, 1967). Both authors describe how it took months to realize that the histories given by the parents were false and that the causal relationship to physical abuse or neglect was present at the outset. Koel (1969) has suggested that failure to thrive and baby battering are on a continuum and Bullard *et al.* (1967) have described 41 infants with failure to thrive whose parents neglected to feed them. Helfer and Pollock (1968) have also described how abused children frequently have 'the added problem of moderate-to-severe malnutrition which often complicates therapy'.

Leonard, Rhymes and Solnit (1966) in their study of 13 infants with failure to thrive, unexplained by organic disease, found the mothers to be lacking in self-esteem and unable to assess their baby's needs and their own work realistically. 'Each can be said to be failing to thrive as a mother and to need nurturing herself to promote her capacity and ability to nurture her baby.'

Adelson (1963) has described 'Homicide by Starvation' as a nutritional variant of baby battering, and Pickel, Anderson and Holliday (1970) reported three cases of hypernatremic dehydration following periodic water deprivation by psychotic mothers.

Dine (1965) has reported an unusual variant of child abuse, by describing a child who presented with bizarre neurological signs; the mother had given this child her own tranquillizer (perphenazine). Griffiths (1974), has had experience of a similar case, but here the mother continued to administer the tranquillizer while the child was still in hospital. Joos (1969) has mentioned that child abuse in a very subtle form is encountered almost daily by the paediatric allergist when he sees children suffering from severe allergic rhinitis or asthma, in whom environmental allergens, such as household pets, play a prominent role. 'These constantly present allergens, despite accumulated evidence showing their cause and effect relationship to the allergic disease are never removed from the home. They remain even in the face of repeated explanations on the part of the physician' (Joos, 1969).

The medical aspects of the battered child syndrome are seen, therefore, to denote a situation ranging from deprivation of food, clothing, shelter and parental love, to incidences where children are physically abused and maltreated by an adult. This may result in obvious physical trauma to the child and frequently death. The degree of association between these various manifestations will be described later.

Chapter 4

Demographic Characteristics

SOCIAL MANIFESTATIONS

Once radiologists and paediatricians had identified parental abuse as a possible cause of serious physical injuries of children and had developed diagnostic case-finding procedures, social workers in children's hospitals became concerned with the implications of this phenomenon for their practice (Gil, 1970). Elizabeth Elmer at the Children's Hospital in Pittsburgh was among the first to discuss this subject. She noted the difficulties professionals had in maintaining an objective and helpful attitude towards those parents who abused their children and drew attention to society's repugnance for the phenomenon. She regarded this as an important factor in the reluctance of many physicians to accept the diagnostic impressions of radiologists (Elmer, 1960).

Complications inherent in comprehensive, interdisciplinary case management of battered children were discussed in a paper by Helen Boardman of the Children's Hospital in Los Angeles (Boardman, 1962). The reluctance of baby batterers to admit attacks on their children, their tendency to repeat such attacks when children were returned home after hospitalization, and the difficulties in obtaining legal evidence in such cases were viewed by Boardman and her medical colleagues as sources of complications in treatment and case management. Despite such complications the staff of the Los Angeles Children's Hospital attempted to develop co-operative, interdisciplinary procedures to provide treatment and services for abused children. Because the child's parents were thought to be in need of protection from the consequences of their uncontrolled behaviour, similar services were provided for the parents.

Kempe *et al.* (1962) reported a high incidence of divorce, separation and unstable marriage as well as minor criminal offences in their sample. Their battered babies were young, often under 1 year of age and in many of the families children were born in rapid succession. Often one child would be singled out for injury and that child was usually unwanted. Over the next decade several authors reported that they supported these findings (Schloesser, 1964; Cameron, Johnson and Camps, 1966; Helfer and Pollock, 1968; Elmer and Gregg, 1967; Johnson and Morse, 1968; Birrell and Birrell, 1968; Ebbin *et al.*, 1969; Skinner and Castle, 1969; Gregg and Elmer, 1969). By way of contrast Steele and Pollock (1968) described baby batterers as representing a 'random cross-section of the general population'. Helfer and Pollock's (1968) comments in this connection are also particularly interesting:

> 'It is probable that if the true figures of child abuse were available, we would see no difference in incidence on a racial, religious, economic or educational basis. However, from the reports that reach the literature it appears that parents who batter children come from the poor and minority groups of our society, primarily because most of these reports originate from large communities or university hospitals serving these classes. In our experience, all cultural, educational, economic and racial backgrounds are represented.'

In 1961 the American Academy of Paediatrics, conducted a symposium on the problem of child abuse under Kempe's direction. The purpose was to plan steps aimed at reducing the prevalence of physical abuse. The conference which was held under the auspices of the U.S. Children's Bureau, recommended the drafting of a model child-abuse reporting statute in all American states (*The Abused Child,* 1963). These efforts were highly successful, for by June 1967 every state in the United States had adopted laws that required or recommended physicians and others to report suspected battered baby cases to appropriate law enforcement or welfare authorities. Such legislation also freed those reporting from civil and criminal liability. One legal authority has commented that 'few legislative proposals in the history of the United States had been so widely adopted in so little time' (Paulsen, 1966).

Merrill (1962) published findings from a study undertaken by the Massachusetts Society for the Prevention of Cruelty to Children. This study examined the cases of 180 abused children from 115 families who had been reported to the agency in 1960. The median age of the children was 7 years. The families of the children were found to suffer from a variety of interpersonal difficulties and were not integrated into their communities. The parents revealed a wide range of personality disorders, and their relationships with the children whom they had abused were severely disturbed. Frequently one specific child in a family appeared to be singled out as a victim.

Another study published at about the same time was a nationwide press survey conducted by Vincent de Francis for the Children's Division of the American Humane Association (de Francis, 1963). During 1962, the Association collected press reports on 662 cases of child abuse, including 178 fatalities. Over 70 per cent had been abused by their parents and fathers were responsible for the more severe injuries. Abuse by fathers resulted primarily from uncontrolled outbursts while disciplining the child. Maternal abuse tended to result from the mother's deep-seated emotional problems. Most families seemed affected by a wide range of internal problems, and most parents seemed emotionally immature. In about 20 per cent of the families there was no father living at home.

The American Humane Association (1963) shortly after publishing this report issued its own guidelines for legislation concerning mandatory reporting of baby battering. These were similar to the Children's Bureau recommendations that the police should receive reports of child abuse; the Humane Association recommended that reports should be made to child protective agencies.

Studies by social workers of characteristics of abusive parents and abused children and of differences between them and neglectful parents and their children continued to be published throughout the 1960s; Young (1964), published a study of 142 cases known to several child protective agencies. Nurse (1964), reported her findings following an intensive study of 20 abusive families known to the juvenile court in New York City, and Elizabeth Elmer and her medical colleagues (Mc Henry, Girdany and Elmer, 1963) published the results of a longitudinal clinical and medical–social investigation of 50 abusive families known to the Children's Hospital in Pittsburgh. All these studies found qualitative differences between abusive and non-abusive parents, and also suggested that many abusive parents had been maltreated by their own parents during childhood. These authors in addition to supporting the findings of Kempe *et al.* (1962), mentioned that social and economic stress, lack of immediate support from extended families, social isolation, high mobility and unemployment were important factors in baby batterers.

Chesser (1952), some 15 years earlier had made similar observations. He reported that cruelty to children was related to deep-seated psychological deviations among the perpetrators, which could often be traced to physical and mental cruelty by their own parents.

In 1963, Bryant and colleagues analysed 134 cases known to the Massachusetts Society for the Prevention of Cruelty to Children. No association was found between social class, intelligence and abuse. In 86 per cent, the children's injuries were inflicted by the natural parents.

Most of the authors in the foregoing review also pointed out that although the socially and economically deprived segments of the community generally contain a high degree of the kinds of stress factors found in baby battering families the great majority of deprived families do not abuse their children.

The following section reviews several studies that have quantified their data concerning certain key demographic characteristics of battered children and their parents. These include: sex and age distribution, ethnic and religious backgrounds and socio-economic status. The findings from these and other reports will be discussed later in the light of some results from this study.

SEX DISTRIBUTION

Battered Children

Simons *et al.* (1966) studied 313 children reported in New York City during the first year of mandatory reporting (1964–1965). Fifty-four per cent of the battered children were girls. Kroeger (1965), in studying a selected sample of abused children known to Chicago hospitals found that 57.7 per cent were boys. Skinner and Castle (1969) observed that the ratio of boys to girls was 3:2 and in Lukianowicz's (1971) sample of 24 battered children the ratio was 2:1.

Gil (1968*b*) also found that slightly more boys than girls were battered, especially among the children whose injuries were fatal (53 per cent of boys to 39 per cent of girls). Analyses of the sex distribution of the different age groups revealed, however, (Gil, 1970) that although boys outnumbered girls in every age group below 12, they were outnumbered by girls among the teenage victims of child abuse. Gil viewed these changes in sex distribution of victims of child abuse during different stages of childhood and adolescence as a reflection of culturally-determined child-rearing attitudes. His opinion is summarized below:

> 'Girls tend to be viewed as more conforming than boys throughout childhood, and physical force tends to be used less frequently in rearing them. However, during stages of sexual maturation, parental anxieties concerning their daughters' heterosexual relationships lead to increasing restrictions, intensified conflicts and increasing use of physical force in asserting parental control. With respect to boys the pattern seems different,

> physical force tends to be used more readily throughout childhood to assure conformity. During adolescence, however as physical strength of boys increases and often matches or even surpasses their parents' strength, the use of physical force in disciplining boys tends to diminish.'

Parents of Battered Children

Simons *et al.* (1966) reported that more women than men were involved as perpetrators and suggested that perpetrators of either sex are more likely to abuse children of their own sex than of the opposite sex. Gil (1968*b*), found that among those parents who had confessed, more women than men were involved in fatal incidents than in non-fatal incidents of baby battering (53 per cent and 45 per cent respectively). He suggested that this was possibly related to the fact that women have a larger part than men in the care of their children.

In Lukianowicz's (1971) sample, 14 mothers battered the child and in two cases it was the father. In a further two cases both parents battered the child, 'although the fathers did it only on their wives' instigation'. Lukianowicz also observed that in all cases the fathers apparently endorsed the aggressive and cruel behaviour of their spouses, or attempted to deny any maltreatment. In three cases the fathers blamed the children as being difficult, stubborn, restless and noisy. By way of contrast Skinner and Castle (1969), found that 56 per cent were mothers and 44 per cent were fathers. Among Bennie and Sclare's (1969) group of 10 child batterers, seven were the mothers of the children. All these studies seem to suggest, therefore, that the general trend is a predominance of battering mothers.

AGE DISTRIBUTION

Battered Children

Many authors have commented on the young age of battered children. Schloesser (1964), found in a study of 85 cases, that 70 per cent were under 3 years of age and 32 per cent were under 6 months. McHenry, Girdany and Elmer (1963), in their sample of 50 cases of multiple skeletal trauma, noted that 60 per cent of the children were under nine months old when battered. Boardman's (1962) sample of 12 cases were all under 3·5 years old, and de Francis (1963) noted that 56 per cent were under 4 years old. Simons *et al.* (1966) found that 28 per cent were under 1 year, 41 per cent were between 1 and 5 years, 23 per cent were between 5 and 10 years and 8 per cent were older than 10 years. Similar results were reported by Kroeger (1965).

Lukianowicz (1971) found the mean age to be 19 months but observed that 'all these children were hated by their mothers almost from the day they were born, and some even before they were born'. Elmer (1963) and Boardman (1962), reported that over 50 per cent of their sample were less than 1 year old. By way of contrast Gil (1970) found that over 75 per cent of his sample were over 2 years of age and nearly 50 per cent were over 6 years. Nearly 20 per cent were teenagers. The age distribution was similar for all ethnic groups.

The finding of many of these studies whereby battered children are very young, may have resulted from bias in the selection and composition of study groups. Many of the above studies were conducted in hospital settings where because of the function of the setting, more severely battered children are seen. Indeed the possibility that younger and more severely injured children are over-represented in samples of battered children selected from hospital populations will be a factor that will be explored later.

Parents of Battered Children

Lukianowicz (1971) found the mean age of mothers to be 22 years with a range of 18–34 years. For fathers, the mean was 24 years with a range of 19–35 years. He concluded that it was mostly young and often emotionally immature parents who battered children. Skinner and Castle (1969) reported a similar age distribution and found that natural fathers were slightly older (mean age 25 years) than substitute fathers (mean age 23 years). Simons *et al.* (1966) found a similar age range in the mothers of 313 abused children; over 35 per cent of them were less than 25 years old and more than 60 per cent were less than 35 years of age. De Francis (1963) reported similar figures.

Gil (1968*b*) has provided a detailed breakdown of the age distribution of perpetrators and suspected perpetrators, nearly 70 per cent of whom were under 30 years old. Gil (1970), has also provided data on the mean age distribution of parents or parent substitutes who did not necessarily confess to baby battering. Among this group 57 per cent of mothers were under 30 years and the corresponding figure for fathers was 37 per cent. Gil's (1970) findings are in striking contrast to his earlier results, and though he does not offer an explanation for the different distributions his concluding comments are nevertheless interesting:

> 'This age distribution does not support the observation of many earlier studies of physically abused children and their families, according to which the parents tend to be extremely young.'

ETHNIC CHARACTERISTICS

Information on ethnic characteristics of battered children is limited. Schloesser (1964) found that battered children did not differ in racial background from the general population. By way of contrast, Simons *et al.* (1966) found that among their sample of 313 children, nearly half (48 per cent) were non-White. Gil (1970) has reported that non-Whites were over-represented to a significant extent; one third (38 per cent) of his sample were non-White. More specifically, of the 1380 children of the sample cohort 39 per cent were White, 46 per cent Negro, 1 per cent American Indian, 7 per cent Puerto Rican, 4 per cent Mexican, 1 per cent Asian and 3 per cent were from other ethnic groups. Perpetrators tended to be of the same race as the children they battered (Gil, 1968*b*).

Gil (1970) is one of the few authors who has discussed the possible reasons for the over-representation of non-Whites. Because his comments will be compared later with some results from this study, it is necessary to provide a summary of his opinions:

> 'Some of the observed over-representation seems to be a function of discriminating attitudes and practices on the part of reporting sources with respect to minority groups . . . The higher reporting rate for non-Whites (may possibly) reflect a real, higher incidence rate of child abuse among ethnic minority groups. Such a higher incidence rate among non-Whites is not unexpected in view of the higher incidence among them of socio-economic deprivation, fatherless homes, and large families, all of which were found . . . to be strongly associated with child abuse. Since different ethnic groups may differ in child rearing practices, the possibility cannot be ruled out that such differences between Whites and non-Whites could be a contributing factor to the observed differences in reporting laws.'

Gil (1970) has also made the interesting suggestion, that ethnically linked differences in using physical force in child rearing may reflect the violence experienced by non-White minorities over many generations in American society.

RELIGION

Information on the religious background of battered children is even more limited than information on their racial background. The religious denominations of 290 families investigated by Simons *et al.* (1966) were as follows; Roman Catholics 44 per cent, Protestants 38 per cent, and other religions 5 per cent (13 per cent of the sample did not report a religion). Gil's (1970) study showed, however, that the religious distribution corresponded closely to the religious distribution of the United

States population. His sample comprised the following; 62 per cent Protestants and other non-Roman Catholic Christians, 26 per cent Roman Catholics, 1 per cent Jewish, 2 per cent other religions, and unknown affiliations 10 per cent. Perpetrators tended to be of the same religious background as the children whom they abused (Gil, 1968*b*).

Lukianowicz's (1971) sample were predominantly Church of Ireland members and a relatively small number were Roman Catholics, but because of the small numbers involved he could not justify any valid conclusions. The contradictory findings of these authors seem to suggest therefore, that religion as such is of little significance in child battering.

SOCIO-ECONOMIC STATUS

Simons *et al.* (1966) reported that nearly half (47 per cent) of their sample of battering parents received financial assistance from the New York Department of Welfare. The proportion was greater (58 per cent) among the non-White parents.

Gil (1970) found that the occupational status of his sample of baby batterers corresponded to their low educational status. A high proportion of the fathers were unemployed and the income of their families was low. Such adversities were worse for non-White groups. Baby batterers also showed a high degree of social mobility. Skinner and Castle's (1969) study also revealed that such parents were extremely mobile 'showing flight as a characteristic of family mobility'.

Lukianowicz's (1971) sample were found predominantly among the lower social classes; 94 per cent were in social classes III, IV and V. This confirmed the findings of an earlier paper (Lukianowicz, 1969). In Skinner and Castle's (1969) study, all parents belonged to social classes III, IV and V. However, in the U.S.A. several authors (Steele and Pollock, 1968; Helfer and Pollock, 1968; Gil, 1968*b*) regard the phenomenon as not being limited to the lower socio-economic groups of the population. The opinion of Oettinger (1968) (though based on little firm evidence) summarizes the current attitude in America to demographic characteristics:

> 'The fact is that some people of every socio-economic, educational, religious and geographical background in our society continue to abuse their children.'

EPIDEMIOLOGICAL STUDIES

The finding and interpretations of medical, psychiatric and social welfare investigations concerning physical abuse of children presented so far in this chapter were derived from observations on relatively small and unrepresentative study samples in specialized settings such as children's hospitals, courts, psychiatric clinics and children's protective services. With the enactment of legislation concerning the reporting of physical abuse of children during the 1960s in America, a source for obtaining data on large numbers of abused children became available for the first time, and research began to shift from clinical studies toward large-scale surveys and epidemiological studies. This shift resulted in certain advantages but also in shortcomings in terms of reliability and validity of research findings. The basis for sample selection was broadened considerably, yet samples of abused children derived through official reporting mechanisms were not necessarily free from systematic bias. Moreover, the detailed observations possible in clinical studies tended to be sacrificed in large scale epidemiological surveys.

Some of the differences in findings and interpretations revealed in the foregoing review were clearly due to differences in the definitions used by various investigators in their sample selection. This particular difficulty continued to haunt designers of large scale epidemiological surveys.

Simons *et al.* (1966), of the School of Public Health and Administrative Medicine at Columbia University, were the first to undertake an epidemiological study of baby battering. Summarizing their findings they state that:

> 'Identification of abused children has assumed new significance with the passage of state laws requiring medical reporting of child abuse incidents. An epidemiologic study of 313 cases registered in New York City during the first year following the 1964 legislation demonstrated a broad spectrum of abuse patterns with a wide range of physical injuries. A strikingly high proportion of the reported children came from multi-problem families where the interplay of mental, physical and environmental stresses could not be ignored as etiologic factors, and where the abused acts appeared chiefly as late indicators of serious family difficulties.'

Following the enactment of reporting legislation, other studies (State of Illinois, 1966; Siker, 1967; State of Maryland, 1968) were published. The findings also revealed a different picture of battering families from those that had emerged as a result of clinical reports and corresponded closely with Simons' (1966) study.

Of the studies surveying the demographic characteristics of families in which child abuse had occurred, the most extensive in scope was the national survey undertaken by Gil (1968*a*, 1968*b*, 1969, 1970). He explored the propensity of the American population to inflict physical injury upon a child by means of a set of questions that funneled the issue down to the individual respondent. Nearly 60 per cent of his sample viewed baby battering 'as an almost normal occurrence', in the course of caring for a child. When the question of propensity was focused directly on the respondent rather than on the population at large, 75 per cent of the sample reported they 'could never injure a child'. Only 20 per cent of the sample considered themselves 'at risk of physically injuring a child some time'. Respondents were next asked how close they came to injuring a child in their care; 15.9 per cent admitted they 'could hardly refrain from injuring a child'.

Gil also reported that baby battering was concentrated among the socio-economically-deprived segments of the population. For Gil, the underlying cause of child abuse in the U.S.A. is the cultural attitude that permits the use of physical force in child rearing. Because he found that the socio-economically-deprived relied more heavily on physical force in their child rearing, he recommended educational efforts aimed at gradually changing this cultural attitude and the establishment of clear cut prohibitions against the use of such physical force. He regarded this educational effort as likely to produce the strongest possible reduction in the incidence and prevalence of physical abuse of children.

While Gil accepted that various forms of physical, social, intellectual and psychological deviance existed among the caretakers and their families, he regarded child abuse as ultimately the result of chance environmental factors. Gil also stressed that the solution to the problem of baby battering rested with a global control of environmental factors. In order to achieve his ultimate objective of reducing 'the general level of violence, and the raising of the general level of human well-being throughout . . . society . . . ', Gil (1969) suggested the following measures which are summarized below.

(1) The elimination of poverty from the midst of America's affluent society.

(2) Prevention and alleviation of deviance and pathology by providing community resources.

(3) Reduction of the numbers of unwanted children by liberalizing laws concerned with therapeutic abortion and the availability of comprehensive family planning programmes.

(4) In preparation for marriage and family life, educational and counselling programmes with the state school system.

(5) The promotion and assurance of maximum feasible physical and mental health for every citizen by a comprehensive, high-quality national health service.

(6) A reduction of environmental stresses in family life by providing a wide range of social services.

(7) Assistance to those families and children who cannot live together because of severe relationship problems and a community-based system of social services.

A number of authors, however, explicitly caution against viewing baby battering as solely a function of educational, occupational, economic or social stress (Adelson, 1961; Kempe *et al.*, 1962; Helfer and Pollock, 1968; Elmer, 1967; Paulson and Blake, 1967; Kempe, 1968; Fontana, 1968; Holter and Friedman, 1968; Steele and Pollock, 1968; Silver, Dublin and Lourie, 1969*a*; Allen, Ten Bensel and Raile, 1969). These authors also agree that raising the general education and financial level of families that are socio-economically deprived is of long-range value in lessening the prevalence of child abuse. They have also pointed to psychological factors within the parents themselves as of prime importance in the aetiology of baby battering. They regard child abuse as stemming from a defect in character leading to lack of inhibition in expressing frustration and other impulsive behaviour. Socio-economic factors sometimes place added stress on the basic weakness in personality structure, but these factors are not of themselves sufficient or necessary causes of abuse.

While one must praise Gil's studies, and his ultimate objective of reducing violence in society there still remains the problem, insoluble at the demographic level, of why some parents batter their children, while others under the same stress factors do not.

Chapter 5

Incidence

INTRODUCTION

Despite increasing awareness, the frequency of the syndrome is not known. The true incidence of child abuse is not available since many cases are not reported or go unrecognized (Helfer and Pollock, 1968). Indeed Gil (1968*b*) has stated that 'readers . . . may be discouraged to learn how little is known about incidence rates and distribution patterns of child abuse'.

This chapter critically reviews the literature on incidence rates available from the U.S.A., Canada and Great Britain, and presents some new data from this study relevant to the problem.

INCIDENCE IN U.S.A. AND CANADA

Conservative estimates have indicated that child abuse in the U.S.A. is so significant that it represents one of the most serious problems confronting the physician who cares for children (Helfer and Pollock, 1968). In 1966, 10 000–15 000 children in the U.S.A. were severely injured by non-accidental means. It is estimated that 5 per cent of these children were killed and 25–30 per cent permanently injured. Helfer's comments (Helfer and Pollock, 1968; Helfer, 1968) place the problem in perspective:

> 'These instances are more significant statistically than the problems and complications associated with common childhood diseases such as measles, mumps and chickenpox . . . To the best of our knowledge at least 250 children are injured in a non-accidental manner for every million population in urban areas. Unless these families are recognized

early and some form of family-centred therapy instituted, approximately 2–3 per cent of these children will be killed each year and 30 per cent of the younger ones will receive permanent physical injury or brain damage.'

Zalba (1966, 1967) has estimated that there are between 200 000 and 250 000 children in the U.S.A. needing protection against serious physical abuse and Gil (1968*b*), has shown that 3–4 per cent of the adults in the U.S.A. personally know of a case of child abuse or neglect. Kempe (1971) suggested that roughly 25 per cent of all fractures seen in the first 2 years of life are due to the battered child syndrome and that '10–15 per cent of all trauma seen in children under 3 years of life were found to be due to this syndrome quite regardless of the history given or the social class of the parents'.

In contrast with these alarming estimates Gil obtained reports from every state government throughout the U.S.A. on every legally reported incident during 1967 and 1968 – a total of 20 500 cases, 12 600 of which involved physical abuse. Gil (1970) suggested that the root cause of child battering is the culturally-approved use of physical force in child rearing, which is endemic in American society, and especially among its poor and uneducated segments and among large, unbroken families.

Gil's comments from an earlier article, Gil (1969), are also interesting:

'Although no claim can be made that the nationwide survey uncovered the true incidence rate of physical abuse of children, it seems clear nevertheless, that the magnitude of the phenomenon has been exaggerated. Six thousand reported cases of physical abuse per year in a nation of 200 million, in spite of under reporting, do not constitute a major social problem, at least in relative terms, tragic as every single incident may be . . . If then the 6000 reported cases represent as a group the more severe segment of the physical abuse spectrum, it follows that in qualitative terms, physical abuse is by and large not very serious as reflected by the data on the extent and types of injury suffered by the children in the study cohort. The classical "battered child" syndrome is a relatively infrequent occurrence. Even if allowance is made for the gross under reporting of fatalities, physical abuse cannot be considered a major killer and maimer of children.'

Gil's report aroused immediate debate and was discussed at length in the correspondence columns of '*Pediatrics*', during 1970. Fontana's (1970) reply provided further information on the incidence of the problem:

'Gil has stated and we agree, that the reported cases of child abuse he has studied constitute only a small part of the total child abuse incidence.

In New York State alone, it is estimated that this past year over 2000 cases of child abuse will have been reported to the child protective agencies in the state — $\frac{1}{3}$ of the total numbers reported by Gil as a nationwide figure . . . In New York Foundling Hospital, at any one time, we have over 300 children — a great majority of these children have been neglected and abused at the hands of their own parents. Another, 1300 children are in foster homes. This is only one child caring institution in one city. At St. Vincent's Hospital and Medical Center of New York, at least 2 or 3 children who have been abused or neglected are seen every month . . . Gil's comments serve to confuse and distort the true nature of this pediatric entity . . . (He) has stated that 'the classical battered child syndrome is a relatively infrequent occurrence'. I am sure that his presence in any of the pediatric emergency units of any large hospital in this country will temper and correct this impression based on paper reports.'

Helfer (1970) was also highly critical of Gil's study.

'I am deeply concerned over Dr. Gil's report on his survey of child abuse. My concern covers all facets of his study; the definition of physical abuse; the use of reports from 1967 which was, for many states the first or second year of their reporting law; setting out to count a certain medical–social problem; and becoming lost in the forest of poverty and hunger of children and the willingness to move from quantitative to the qualitative . . . and reaching conclusions that cannot be supported by the data.

Although the true incidence of child abuse will likely never be known, a realistic assessment can now be made from the current reporting rates in Denver and New York City . . . The number of reports in these two cities ranges between 175 and 225 per million population per year. Were other cities to give as much effort to this problem as have Denver and New York City, the number of cases reported per year in the United States would reach between 30 000 and 50 000 . . . this is still only the tip of the abnormal child rearing iceberg.'

Helfer concluded his criticism of Gil's report by expressing the hope that further research would clarify our understanding of the child rearing processes and that this would lead to meaningful therapeutic approaches.

Mary Van Stolk (1972) believes that the statistics, derived from Denver, Colorado, and mentioned above, apply equally to Canada. Using a slightly more conservative estimate of 225 cases per million population, Van Stolk concluded that 1718 injuries and 34–52 fatalities from child abuse can be expected each year in Ontario. Such figures are considerably in excess of the officially reported cases. Because the Children's Aid Societies have no statutory obligation to report such cases to a Central Register she has argued that the official figures underestimate the true incidence. The Canadian Government is currently assessing whether mandatory reporting will improve upon existing knowledge concerning incidence rates (Greenland, 1973).

In Ontario, Children's Aid Societies reported 1603 cases to the Central Register during the 5 year period from 1966 to 1970 (Greenland, 1973). These 1603 cases involved approximately 1800 children – an average of 360 per year. In the same period, 1966–1970, according to the Coroner's office, physical abuse or criminal negligence was the probable cause of 40 infants deaths. Not all of these cases were known to the local Children's Aid Society. Greenland (1973) also showed that there was considerable variation in the number of cases reported by Children's Aid Societies in Canada and demonstrated that Societies used different definitions of child abuse when reporting a case to the Registrar; some for example included cases of incest and sexual assault while others reported medically diagnosed cases of physical abuse. Britain has no law that governs statutory notification of battered baby cases. Nevertheless, several authors have provided estimates of the incidence of the problem and their studies are briefly reviewed in the following section.

INCIDENCE IN GREAT BRITAIN

The true incidence of the syndrome in Great Britain is not known. Chesser (1952) has generally estimated that between 6 and 7 per cent of all children are at some time during their life 'so neglected or ill-treated . . . as to require the help of the N.S.P.C.C.' Kempe, in the 1970 Windermere Lecture (Kempe, 1971) has remarked that:

> 'For 500 000 new babies born each year in Great Britain there may be, 3000 cases each year of which half will be significantly injured and the other half seriously deprived. . . '

In West Germany the number of prosecutions for parental maltreatment is between 300 and 400 per year, but this represents only a small proportion (5 per cent), of all cases of parental abuse (Köttgen, 1967; Lukianowicz, 1971). Arguing on the basis that West Germany has a population almost identical in size to that of Great Britain, Lukianowicz (1971), has calculated that there are 8000 children battered each year in West Germany and that a similar number occurs in Great Britain.

Hall (1975), Consultant in Charge of the Emergency and Accident Department at Preston Royal Infirmary, has also estimated the incidence of the battered baby syndrome in Great Britain based on the numbers he has personally seen:

> 'In 1970, 1971 and 1972 a total of 29 definite cases including five deaths were seen. The average incidence per annum is 9.6 per cent and the

mortality rate is 17.2 per cent. Fifteen million patients are treated annually in the emergency departments of the country. In Preston 34 000 patients were treated in 1972. The incidence of these cases is 1 in 3400 of the attendances at the Preston Emergency Department. If this is related to a national incidence of fifteen million attendances per annum, then it might be expected that 4400 such children would be seen throughout the country every year.'

A mortality rate of 17·2 per cent would give a national mortality rate of 757 per annum. This latter figure is approximately 50 per cent of the national death rate from leukaemia in children up to the age of 3 years.

Hall has estimated that morbidity may be in the order of 10 per cent since head injuries feature largely in the medical records and sub-dural haematomata are a common cause of death. Because such cases are referred to a neurosurgical unit he has remarked 'that social investigation is unlikely to be carried out . . . ' and that this particularly occurs when the specialist unit is not part of the hospital which originally received the case. Lack of communication to other agencies resulted in the death of one of his patients.

Oliver *et al.* (1974) have attempted to ascertain the prevalence of child abuse in North East Wiltshire. Using very strict criteria of baby battering (which thus excluded minor injuries) they collected a total of 38 children over a period of 7 years (1965–1971). These children came from 34 families; four families each contributing two children. A further 20 children were collected in a period of 18 months from January 1972 to June 1973. These authors reported on the rate of severe abuse as follows:

'The total rate for the whole seven year period was 2.6 per thousand children under four years old. It was slightly higher in males than in females, the difference being almost wholly accounted for by males first assaulted at ages 2 and 3 years. The rate for children under one year was 8.5 per thousand.'

Following a year of educative activity with the professions involved, a further 20 children were ascertained over a separate period of 18 months giving an annual rate of 0.91 per thousand children under 4 years of age; an increase of 2.5 times. In a later section of their report the authors commented that the rate of 0.91 new cases referred per thousand children under 4 years old 'was likely to be an underestimate and . . . that a rate of 1 per thousand seemed reasonable'.

'This would mean about 3000 children aged 0–3 years should be referred every year in England and Wales as a whole , . . the death rate might be about 0.1/1000 (300 per year in England and Wales) and this would be approximately one to two thirds the rate for deaths from trauma in this age group, and about 2–2.5 per cent of all deaths in children aged 0–3.'

The authors of this very detailed report, which confined its attention to children under 4 years of age, readily admit that their figures are modest estimates only, but are of the opinion that the likely rate of severe attacks on children under 5 years of age would be 10/100 000 population. Projecting their figures to the country as a whole, the minimum rate of severe attacks on children under 5 years of age would be 2450 per annum. These figures are higher than Kempe's (1971) estimate of 1500 cases of battered babies per year for Britain.

Published reports dealing with, or touching upon, the prevalence of child abuse have accepted that even the most severe forms of active battering of very young children are not often recognized by doctors, social workers or other professional people (Holter and Friedman, 1968; Silver, Dublin and Lourie, 1969*a*; Skinner and Castle, 1969; Cameron, 1972; Jackson, 1972). Estimates of the extent of child abuse have been gross underestimates and have been recognized as such (Kempe, 1971; Okell, 1971; Jackson, 1972; Colclough, 1972).

Figures for 1967 from the Registrar General (1969) detail a total of 71 deaths to children under the age of 5 years due to 'homicide and injury purposely inflicted by other persons'; 43 of these deaths occurred in the first year of life. Other sources (Central Health Services Council, 1970) suggest that there could be some 40 infant deaths per annum from wilful violence, in the first year of life.

THE NEED FOR RELIABLE STATISTICS

Table 1 shows the number of deaths due to 'homicide and injury purposely inflicted' and 'undetermined, accidental or purposely inflicted injuries' based on the Registrar General's causes of death between 1968 and 1971 (Registrar General, 1970, 1971, 1972*a, b*, 1973).

TABLE 1
Deaths in Children 0–4 Years Old, Due to 'Homicide and Injury Purposely Inflicted' and 'Undetermined Accidental or Purposely Inflicted Injuries'

Cause of death	*1968*	*1969*	*1970*	*1971*
Homicide and injury purposely inflicted	82	77	76	68
Undetermined, accidental or purposely inflicted injuries	49	51	31	28

Though the time interval is small (figures are unobtainable prior to 1967), these statistics at first glance suggest a steady decline in the number of officially reported battered baby cases. Considering that other violent crimes have shown a steady increase in the past few years (Walker, 1971), the reliability of the official statistics representing the true incidence of the problem may be questioned. Such cases which are reported may thus only represent the tip of the iceberg.

Diggle and Jackson (1973) have recently proposed that a realistic and accurate assessment of the scale and nature of the battered baby problem can be made by a computer-based system working initially at Local Authority, Regional and eventually National level. They failed to mention, however, that several Local Authorities have already established confidential central registers concerning such children. Furthermore, medical personnel presently have at their disposal a 'Request for Information Form' that provides information similar to the more elaborate scheme they propose (Smith, 1972, 1973).

The use of these forms was assessed during the course of this study. The relevant form was made available at casualty departments and paediatric wards throughout the region and doctors were instructed that when confronted with a case, they should complete this form and forward it to the Social Services Department. Following this they received a prompt reply informing them whether the child had been previously battered or suspected of being battered. A list of the names, telephone numbers and addresses of those previously involved with the child were also supplied. This procedure was approved by the Medical Defence Union as involving no breach of confidentiality.

Nevertheless of 134 cases that came to the authors' attention, in only 33.3 per cent was the form completed. Perhaps, therefore, Diggle and Jackson's confidential files might be used if they were made available at paediatric hospitals rather than social services departments. However, it may still be erroneous to assume that their scheme will necessarily provide reliable statistics because there are still likely to be a number of doctors who fail to provide their computer with information. To rely on the discretion of casualty officers and others to provide relevant information seems rather optimistic in the light of experience. As mentioned previously, even in the U.S.A., where mandatory reporting of battered baby cases has been in existence for a number of years, conflicting estimates still occur. Furthermore, even if reliable statistics were available this does not necessarily imply efficient management of the problem. However, improvement could readily be made if doctors accurately recorded the correct diagnosis on the summary discharge sheet (Smith and Hanson, 1974). This still too rarely occurs.

Diggle and Jackson's computer-based system has recently been adopted on a trial basis in Wiltshire (Oliver, 1974). An evaluation of the success of this scheme in providing accurate statistics on the problem is awaited with interest.

Chapter 6

Psychiatric Aspects: A Review of the Literature

INTRODUCTION

According to Kempe (1970), every parent is a potential 'baby basher'. Fleming (1967), has pointed out that there can be very few parents who, at one time or another, have not been exasperated beyond endurance by the behaviour of their children. Fortunately for most, the expression of their exasperation stops short of real violence. Gil (1970) has argued that anyone can be a child batterer, and that no matter how kind they may appear under normal circumstances, if placed under enough pressure they will batter their children. He has also argued that a certain measure of physical abuse of children is condoned by American culture as a 'normal' aspect of rearing children.

Zalba (quoted in Van Stolk, 1972) commenting on what appears to be a lack of awareness of child abuse asks:

> 'Is there any mother or father who has not been "provoked" almost to the breaking point by the crying, wheedling child? How many parents have not had moments of concern and self-recrimination after having in anger, hit their own child much harder than they expected they would? How many such incidents make a "child abuser" out of a normal parent? There may be a tacit agreement among us not to meddle in each others private matters unless it is simply impossible to ignore the behaviour involved.'

In contrast to these recent views, anthropological evidence (Malinowski, 1927; Mead, 1928; Gorer, 1968) shows that whole civilizations or whole groups of people suffering from extreme stresses, deprivation and frustrations have not and would not lash out at their children.

Van Stolk (1972), has also challenged the belief that child battering in times of stress is normal or human nature.

> 'There is no evidence to indicate that all people are potential child batterers. There is no evidence to support the supposition that given enough pressure, tension and trauma a man or woman will turn upon his or her young child and strike out.'

She has argued convincingly (Van Stolk, 1972), that child battering is abnormal behaviour and should no longer be dismissed as a regrettable but inevitable aspect of human nature. 'Instead the inside mechanisms, as well as the cultural mechanics, which create and maintain a structure of child battering, must be investigated'.

It is not surprising, therefore, that when the literature on the psychiatric aspects of baby batterers is reviewed a diffuse picture emerges.

AN OVERVIEW OF THE PSYCHIATRIC LITERATURE

A number of authors have regarded neurotic or psychotic behaviour as of strong aetiological importance (Woolley and Evans, 1955; Miller, 1959; Platou, Lennox and Beasley, 1964; Greengard, 1964; Cochrane, 1965; Simpson, 1967, 1968). Adelson (1961) and Kaufman (1962) considered that the most violent and abusive parents are schizophrenic. Kempe *et al.* (1962), while accepting that frank psychosis on the part of the parents was responsible for direct murder of children, suggested that most baby batterers, though lacking in impulse control were not severely psychotic. Other authors also supported this view (Laupus, 1966; Wasserman, 1967; Fleming, 1967; Steele and Pollock, 1968). While most authors generally agree that there is a defect in the parents' personality that allows aggressive impulses to be expressed too freely (Kempe *et al.*, 1962; Wasserman, 1967; Steele and Pollock, 1968) disagreement comes in describing the source of the aggressive impulses (Spinetta and Rigler, 1972).

Some authors claim that abuse is a final outburst at the end of a long period of tension (TenHave, 1965; Nomura, 1966), or that it stems from an inability to face life's daily stresses (Heins, 1969). Others claim that abuse stems from deep feelings of inadequacy or from inability to fulfil the parental role (Cohen, Raphling and Green, 1966; Komisaruk, 1966; Silver, 1968; Johnson and Morse, 1968; Steele and Pollock, 1968; Fontana, 1971). Others also describe the parents as immature self-centred and impulse ridden (Ten Bensel, 1963; Jacobziner, 1964; Cochrane, 1965).

Role reversal between the spouses had also been considered a prime factor in the aetiology of baby battering. A home in which the father is unemployed and the mother has taken over the financial responsibility of the family is considered a breeding ground for abuse (Nurse, 1964; Greengard, 1964; Galdston, 1965; Nathan, 1965).

Several authors have also considered that low intelligence among the parents is important (Fisher, 1958; Simpson, 1967, 1968). Zlotnik (quoted in Vesterdal, 1972) found that among a series of 23 adults prosecuted for maltreatment, eight were mentally retarded. He suggested a 'battering parent syndrome' characterized by character deviations such as immaturity, aggressiveness and psychic infantilism. By way of contrast others suggest that baby batterers have normal intelligence (Kempe *et al.*, 1962; Cameron, Johnson and Camps, 1966; Holter and Friedman, 1968*b*; Ounsted, 1968) or range 'from low borderline figures of I.Q.s in the 70's to superior ratings of 130' (Steele and Pollock, 1968).

Some recent studies have also shown that baby battering overlaps with other criminal behaviour (Smith, Hanson and Noble, 1973; Oliver *et al.*, 1974). Smith, Hanson and Noble (1973) have also described a group of baby batterers who were in many ways similar to a group of fathers who killed their children (Scott, 1973) and to Zlotnik's group of Danish parents (quoted in Vesterdal, 1972) convicted of child abuse. Scott (1973), observed that more than 25 per cent of his sample had convictions for juvenile offences and a similar proportion had been convicted for violent offences. Several had been to E.S.N. schools but were not subnormal within the terms of the Mental Health Act, 1959, a finding also observed by others (Oliver and Cox, 1973; Oliver *et al.*, 1974).

Zlotnik (quoted in Vesterdal, 1972) noted that nearly 66.6 per cent of baby batterers had character disorders or constitutional psychopathy which were associated with multiple psychological and social difficulties. Scott (1973) also found that 'no psychiatric diagnoses other than personality disorder can be made, but this exists in 75 per cent of cases. Most cases had high environmental stress and a high degree of personality handicap'.

The following section reviews some of these studies in detail.

A TYPOLOGY OF BABY BATTERERS

Realization that each of the above described characteristics was found to exist in at least some individual circumstances has led some authors to group together certain characteristics in clusters and to evolve a psychodynamic within each cluster.

The first major attempt at a dynamic typology was made by Merrill (1962), who suggested that battering mothers and fathers had three distinct clusters of personality characteristics. A fourth cluster was characteristic of fathers only. Merrill's groups are summarized below.

GROUP 1

These seemed to be beset with continual and pervasive hostility and aggressiveness sometimes focused and sometimes directed at the world in general. This was not a controlled anger and was continually with the parents, with the only stimulation needed for direct expression, being normal daily difficulties. This angry feeling stemmed from conflicts within the parents and was often rooted in their early childhood experiences.

GROUP 2

These were identified by personality characteristics of rigidity, compulsiveness, lack of warmth, lack of reasonableness and lack of pliability in thinking and attitudes. Such parents defended their right to batter their child. The mothers had marked child-rejection attitudes, showed an inability to feel love and protectiveness towards their children. They were concerned with their own pleasures and felt that their children were responsible for many of their troubles. Such parents were extremely compulsive and demanded excessive cleanliness of their children. They had difficulty with verbal expression in relaxing and in exhibiting warmth and friendliness.

GROUP 3

These were characterized by strong feelings of passivity and dependence, and often competed with their own children for the love and attention of their spouses. Many of these parents showed considerable immaturity and were generally depressed, moody, unresponsive and unhappy.

GROUP 4

These included a significant number who were generally young intelligent men with acquired skills who because of some physical disability were now fully or partially unable to support their families. In most of the situations the mothers worked while the fathers stayed home and cared for the children. Their frustrations led to swift and severe punishment and to angry, rigid discipline.

Bryant (1963) has suggested three distinct clusters of parental pathology.

(1) Hostility and aggressiveness, which included parents who appeared to be angry in a continuous and uncontrolled manner. This seemed directly attributable to the parents' early childhood experiences.
(2) Characteristics of rigidity, compulsiveness and lack of warmth. Many had marked attitudes of child rejection and were extremely compulsive in their behaviour.
(3) Those who showed strong feelings of passivity and dependence. These parents competed with their children for the love and attention of their spouses; a general depression being frequently interwoven as part of the personality pattern. Some were still dominated by their families.

Delsordo (1963) reported the findings of a study of 80 cases of abused children who had been reported to the Pennsylvania Society to Protect Children from Cruelty. The purpose of this study was not only to describe the cases but to develop a typology of abusive parents which could guide treatment, and particularly cover the question of whether an abused child should be removed from the parents' custody or remain in their care. Delsordo (1963) identified five types in this study.

(1) Abuse resulting from 'parents' mental illness'.
(2) Abuse as 'an overflow from the parents' aimless way of life'.
(3) 'A non-specific disturbance in the parent resulting in severe battering of the child'.
(4) Abuse due to 'parents' harshness in disciplining children'.
(5) Abuse due to 'parents' misplaced conflicts'.

In spite of its crudeness this typology was useful in practice. Delsordo recommended that children should be removed from their parents' care in the first three types.

Zalba (1967), published a more systematic typology of child abuse based on the locus of the problems and the parents' ability to control abusive behaviour in the future. With slight modifications, however, the typology of Delsordo (1963) and Zalba (1967), can be reduced to Merrill's (1962) categories. The six types identified by Zalba are shown in Table 2.

Zalba suggested that children should not be left in the custody of parents belonging to the first three types, but could be left with

TABLE 2
Classification of Abusive Parents (Zalba, 1967)

Locus of problem	*Parents ability to control abuse*	
	Not able to control	*Able to control*
Personality system	(1) Psychotic parent (2) Pervasively angry and abusive parent (3) Depressive, passive-aggressive parent	
		(4) Cold, compulsive disciplinarian parent
Family system		(5) Impulsive but generally adequate parent with marital conflict
Person-environment or Family-environment system		(6) Parent with identity/role crisis

parents belonging to types 4–6, provided the parents received appropriate treatment.

The use of such typologies seems at first glance to be simple unifying and time saving. However, there has been no evidence to show that such categories or similar clusters are valid or whether they are useful as an aid in the determination of high-risk patients.

This difficulty has recently been pointed out by Schneider, Helfer and Pollock (1972), who for the past several years have attempted 'to design and validate a questionnaire with the goal of uncovering parents who have the potential to abuse their small children'. Rather than relying on a score of a certain level above which an abusive potential is indicated, these researchers looked for the clusters of questions to which potential abusers gave abnormal answers. The principal areas in which the questions clustered were; feelings of loneliness and isolation, expectations for performance of their children, relationships with their own parents and spouse and feelings of anxiety in response to their children's behaviour. Statistical findings from the first pilot study confirmed that abusing parents differ in these areas.

A second study involved a control group of non-abusing parents and their responses to 50 discriminating questions; all the responses were subject to a cluster analysis seeking to group those questions with similar patterns of intercorrelation. Five different personality types emerged; two types of abusing parents exactly fitted the predictions which psychiatrists had made, while two other types denied that they had the expected attitudes in some but not in all the principal prediction areas. These findings were thought to indicate that if enough discriminating questions are asked, in enough areas, an abuser will give a sufficiently abnormal pattern response to permit of his identification.

Schneider, Helfer and Pollock (1972) conclude their preliminary report of this interesting research by placing their findings in perspective:

> 'Only further data analysis will indicate if we have been successful in this extra-ordinarily difficult task of constructing a valid and reliable questionnaire which will be useful in identifying parents who have the potential to abuse small children.'

Unfortunately this questionnaire is still in its developmental stages, has not yet been completely validated, and cannot be used for other than research purposes.

PSYCHODYNAMICS

At a conference held at the University of Colorado School of Medicine in 1966, Galdston, a psychiatrist at the Children's Hospital in Boston, presented the following interpretations of the psychodynamics of baby batterers. He viewed the syndrome as the result of a parents attempt to cope with internal conflict by means of externalization. Table 3 itemizes those factors that Galdston believes collectively disposed a parent to resort to baby battering. He further suggested that such factors spared the parents from the conscious experience of their own intrapsychic stress (Galdston, 1966).

Milowe, a psychiatrist, at the Children's Hospital in Washington D.C., was also a participant in this conference and expressed scepticism (Milowe, 1966) concerning the extent of psychiatric understanding of baby batterers. He was also critical of Galdston's psychodynamic interpretation.

> 'Our information about the personality patterns of parents who batter their children remains largely anecdotal. Similar life circumstances and dynamics coexist in other parents who do not batter their children and we are unable to quantify our studies of the inter-relationship between ego strength, life stress, intensity of sadistic impulses and resultant battering.'

Milowe (1966) was the first to suggest that children themselves may in certain situations contribute to their own abuse. He also pointed to the intergenerational dimension of abusive child rearing problems.

> 'Some of these infants are atypically difficult and irritating children. Some have described a particularly grating quality to their crying; nurses

TABLE 3
Psychodynamics of Baby Batterers (Galdston, 1966)

(1)	Major reliance upon projection as a leading defence against intrapsychic stress. There is a defect in their capacity to test the reality of the child. The child functions as a delusion in what is essentially a transference psychosis.
(2)	A tendency to translate affect states into physical activity without intervention of conscious thought.
(3)	The presence of intolerable self-hatred; This is the 'it', which the parent 'takes out' on the child . . . tries to dispose of . . . by projecting . . . on to the child and exorcising . . . through physical abuse. The child is the scapegoat for the parent's sense of guilt.
(4)	Correspondence of the child by sex, age and position in the family to events in the parent's own life which occasioned . . . great self-hatred . . . It is the presence of the child of a particular sex, age and position which serves as the seed crystal about which the parent's forgotten unwanted emotions threaten to precipitate out of unconscious into awareness.
(5)	Relative lack of available alternative modes of defence against conflict because of environmental factors; poverty, illness, domestic demands, social isolation, housing problems, all can contribute an increment to the likelihood of physical abuse by reducing the availability of alternative modes for discharging intrapsychic tensions.
(6)	Compliance with the act of abuse by the marriage partner due to dependence and reciprocal willingness to support projective defences.
(7)	Relative absence of available authority figures. The deterrent power of grandparents, religious or social authorities as an antidote to idiosyncratic perceptions and eccentric behaviour is seldom available to the abusive parent.

> and social workers have confessed understanding why a parent might batter "THAT CHILD". Indeed, reports confirm that some of these children get battered in sequential foster home placements where no other child has been battered . . . In some families such violence can be traced through at least three generations.'

Henry Makover, a psychiatrist at the Albert Einstein College of Medicine, discussed his observations and psychodynamic interpretations based on experience of battered baby cases which came before the Family Court of New York. He suggested (Makover, 1966), that such cases differed in certain respects from those seen in hospitals and psychiatric clinics:

> 'My observations indicate that overt mental illness, as manifested by psychotic or borderline behaviour, is present more frequently in the parent or parents of the physically abused child than it is in other forms of neglect . . . A high proportion of the families seen show the effects of poverty and overcrowding, and, therefore, social stress is more likely to be present in these cases on the basis of probability alone.'

The following were among the more overt forms of mental illness he encountered: chronic paranoid schizophrenia, psychopathic personality, agitated depression, and particularly unresolved post-partum depression. Alcoholism was also seen but more often cited as a precipitant. Narcotic addiction was infrequent, though it contributed to the neglect of children by draining the families economic reserves. Other forms of mental disorder were, mental retardation, sexual deviance, psychomotor equivalents and an 'unconscious displacement of the spouse or even of the parent's parents'.

Brandt Steele who with Henry Kempe was co-sponsor of this conference also questioned some of the interpretations offered by his psychiatric colleagues (Steele, 1966). Based on intensive studies and treatment of 60 abusive families which he and his colleagues at the University of Colorado had conducted over 4 years, he concluded that the broad range of personality disturbances that had been found in association with baby battering occurred also with persons who did not abuse their children. Thus it was not possible to view these conditions as sufficient causal explanations of child abuse. His comments are interesting:

> 'What provokes child beating? An incredible sense of aloneness, worthlessness and strangely enough desire – desire for the child to take care of the unheeded needs of the attacker's own yesterdays. When the baby cries or when the small child doesn't yield, his caretaker cannot tolerate the feeling provoked within himself. Attack is the only solution this caretaker knows.'

His observations led him to consider that the basic problem was that of a breakdown in 'ability to mother', which he defined as 'the deep, sensitive intuitive awareness of and response to the infant's condition and needs, as well as consideration of the infant's capacity to perform according to his age' (Steele, 1966). Steele and Pollock (1968), in their analysis of the mothering function and its vicissitudes, have also interpreted the neglected child and the infant who fails to thrive as a more passive phenomenon of rejection than that involved in child battering.

Because Steele and Pollock's viewpoint has had considerable influence on management concepts, and because their theories will later be compared with findings from this study, it is necessary at this stage to provide a synopsis of their views.

In their study of 60 families in which significant abuse of children occurred, the parents studied represented a wide range of personality types. There was no one psychiatric diagnosis which was associated with this behaviour and findings of psychosis was rare. They usually showed various combinations of schizoid, hysterical or obsessive-compulsive personality traits and no one type was an indicator of potential child abuse. In their study, all socio-economic levels were represented and most of the parents appeared to be well adjusted members of the community who had a wide range of intelligence quotients, varying from the dull-normal to superior. They asserted that physicians should not be misled by considering that child abuse can occur only in a certain state of society or only in the presence of severe mental illness. They drew attention to two particular psychological circumstances within the family. The first is a particular pattern in which children are perceived and reacted to by the parents. The second is the set of stressful circumstances which brings out and enhances this pattern of parental behaviour.

This pattern of child-rearing encompasses a set of attitudes in which children are expected to satisfy many of the parents' emotional needs. One manifestation of the pattern is an insistence upon a high level of performance from extremely small children. The mother insists on expectations of behaviour from the child far beyond his chronological age. Older children in these families are often very skilled at supplying emotional support for their parents. This pattern goes far beyond the enforcement of strict standards of excellence for the children, because what is actually required of them is that they understand and sympathize with their parents' needs for affection. Although parents exploit their children for many of their own purposes, it appears that this intense need to turn to the child for affection is an important underlying feature of the child-beating parent. If no gratification is received from the child the parent responds with frustration and anger. Clues can be seen in the case of the distraught or upset mother who reacts with anger and anxiety toward the child when he is sick or crying excessively and not responsive to her attempts to comfort him. This behaviour may erupt in violence if followed to an extreme and no one intervenes.

The second set of circumstances is the presence of additional types of stressful situations for the parents. The battering parent often feels unable to receive emotional support from the spouse or other relatives. Because the parents have a large residue of unfulfilled emotional needs themselves they are extremely sensitive to withdrawal of such support from their environment. The young mother who had had a difficult time with her pregnancy and who received little support from her spouse or her family, may see the demands of child-rearing as overwhelming. If the child represents someone to whom she expects to turn, the mother may look toward the child for much of the understanding and support that is lacking in her present situation. It is for this reason, according to Steele and Pollock, that child abuse most frequently occurs at times when the spouse is physically or emotionally absent and no other support is possible for the abusing parent.

By way of contrast, Kaufman (1962), in discussing the personality of baby batterers, asserted the violence they displayed was associated with some type of unreality, and in its most extreme form was associated with a type of schizophrenic process. Although Kaufman went on to state that many of the parents he had seen were not overtly schizophrenic, he also argued that individuals who had episodic outbursts of loss of control, loss of reason and loss of judgement represent a type of schizophrenia:

> 'Attacking a child is a crime of violence, and some of the persons who get so violently out of control may fall into the category of the antisocial schizophrenic.'

Kaufman, also commented on the transmission of the abusive pattern from parents to children and considered the impact such parents had as identification figures for their children. He argued that the antisocial schizophrenic tended to come from disruptive homes where violent abusive parents would demonstrate uncontrolled aggressive behaviour. Such parents were unrelated to the community and had a psychotic core, in that their basic anxieties were related to fears of annihilation, which they handled by externalizing and attacking.

Kaufman does not quote the criteria used in formulating the presence of a schizophrenic process. It is possible that many of the characteristics he described would be regarded as typical of the psychopath by British psychiatrists (Walton and Presly, 1973).

CHILDHOOD EXPERIENCES AND PATTERNS OF CHILD REARING

In 1963, the Child Welfare League of America published a collection of papers entitled '*The Neglected Battered Child Syndrome*' (Morris and Gould, 1963). The subtitle of this pamphlet, '*Role Reversal in Parents*', reflected the attempt of the authors to develop a psychiatric conceptualization of child abuse. Morris, Gould and Matthews (1964) suggested that an abusing parent views his victim not as the child he really is but as his own parent, who has failed, hurt and frustrated him. The abuse is intended for the absent parent, but is displaced and acted out against the helpless present child. The child in such cases is expected by the parent to meet his (the parent's) complex emotional needs, rather than having his needs met by the parent; when the child fails to do so, the frustrated parent, attacks, injures and at times destroys the child. Morris, Gould and Matthews (1964), also explored differences in the behaviour of abusive and non-abusive parents, and of abused and non-abused children. The purpose of these explorations was to provide medical and social-welfare personnel with diagnostic clues that would aid in case finding, in the planning of treatment for individual cases, and in the prevention of re-battering.

Steele and Pollock (1968), have also argued that such parents have a history of having been raised in the same style that they have recreated in the pattern of rearing their own children. They suggest that as infants and children all baby batterers were deprived of basic mothering and of the deep sense of being cared for and cared about from the beginning of their lives. Fontana (1968), also viewed the parents as emotionally crippled because of unfortunate circumstances in their own childhood. Such parents reacted to their children in keeping with their own experiences of loneliness, lack of protection and lack of love.

Several other authors have also suggested that baby batterers prematurely expect and demand a great deal from their children, and show a corresponding disregard for the child's own limited abilities and helplessness (Bain, 1963; Korsch *et al.*, 1965; Helfer and Pollock, 1968; Gregg, 1968; Johnson and Morse, 1968; Hiller, 1969). Wasserman (1967) suggested that such parents not only considered punishment a proper disciplinary measure but strongly defended their right to use physical force. Scott (1973) also found that a fathers' interpretation of his child's behaviour was important and supported Morris and Gould's (1963) claim of 'role reversal'.

Spinetta and Rigler (1972), in reviewing the background experiences of baby batterers, concluded that many abusing parents were themselves raised with some degree of abuse or neglect and that this was responsible for their inappropriate knowledge of child rearing techniques.

> 'Their attitudes, expectations and child rearing techniques set them apart from non-abusive parents. The abusing parents implement culturally accepted norms for raising children with an exaggerated tendency and at an inappropriately early age.'

Gibbens and Walker (1956), in a survey of 32 men and 7 women who had been imprisoned for cruelty to their children, concluded that it was rejection, indifference and hostility in their own childhood that produced cruel parents. Tutuer and Glotzer (1966), studied 10 mothers who had murdered their children and found that all had been reared in an extremely cold and often overtly rejecting environment. Parental figures were either absent or offered little opportunity for healthy identification when present. Komisaruk (1966), found that the emotional loss of a significant parental figure in the early life of battering parents was also important.

Melnick and Hurley (1969), have carried out one of the few systematic and well-controlled studies of baby batterers. They compared two small, socio-economic and racially-matched groups on 18 personality variables, and found, among other things, a probable history of emotional deprivation in the mothers' own upbringing. This caused the mothers to have severely frustrated dependency needs and an inability to empathize with their own children.

Other authors also mention that baby batterers were themselves battered or neglected as children (Easson and Steinhilber, 1961; Kempe *et al.*, 1962; Curtis, 1963; Harper, 1963; McHenry, Girdany and Elmer, 1963; Bryant, 1963; Morris, Gould and Matthews, 1964; Corbett, 1964; Green, 1965; Fairburn and Hunt, 1964; Bleiberg, 1965, Blue, 1965, Wasserman, 1967; Silver, Dublin and Lourie, 1969*b*; Paulson and Blake, 1969). Gluckman (1968), in reviewing the findings of earlier authors, listed 10 differential diagnostic categories. He also argued that the capacity to love is not inherent but must be taught to the child, and that many battering parents were raised without such love and tolerance.

Craft (1969), in describing the background of psychopaths, similarly reported that there is a general tendency for association of parental cruelty and violence to be recapitulated in their children'. Similarly Reiner and Kaufman's (1959) conclusions are also pertinent:

> '(Children who) experienced loss of love . . . are unable as adults to provide a mature and consistent type of parental care for their children, but pass on these elements to them. (Furthermore) such parents have a tendency to subject their own children to similar losses and to experiences that will engender the same attitudes.'

Lukianowicz (1971), described the early childhood experiences of 18 mothers who had battered their children. Five had uneventful but not exactly 'happy' experiences, six were unhappy, three had stressful and three others had indifferent childhoods. No reliable information could be obtained about the childhood experiences of one subject. Lukianowicz (1971), concluded that:

> 'most women in our group had themselves had a rather unhappy and loveless, or traumatic childhood, which seems to have influenced their attitude to their own children, and in some cases also to their husbands'.

Scott (1973), in a study of 29 fathers who had been charged with killing their young child, found that 19 were from punitive backgrounds and 12 of these remembered parental violence (two from their mothers). Five had institutional backgrounds, but 10 were from normal homes.

Scott's comments on the factors contributing to baby battering are interesting:

> 'Two sets of circumstances account for battering by a parent who was well cared for as a child. First it seems that mental immaturity can sometimes exist as a clinical entity independently of mishandling . . . Second, weak husbands who are influenced by stronger and punitive wives, sometimes seem to have battering thrust upon them.'

Scott's (1973) succinct assessment of the early childhood experiences of his group of fathers (which could probably equally be applied to battering mothers), also places the literature on this point in perspective.

> 'It does seem clear, therefore, that occasionally battering can be carried out by a father whose early handling cannot be faulted. Such cases must be contrasted with the common ones in which the aggression seems to be handed on from generation to generation.'

CONCLUSION

Emerging from this chapter is a conglomerate picture of parental motivational and personality factors, with several authors' attempts to cluster the characteristics into a workable unity. One fact of agreement, however, arising from all these studies is that baby batterers have a general defect in character (from whatever source), that allows aggressive impulses to be expressed too freely on a helpless child. The purpose of bringing together the published professional opinions on the psychiatric characteristics of such parents, has been to determine the most commonly held opinions, in order that more systematic testing of hypotheses can be carried out. The generalizations that have been deduced from this literature review will be re-examined later in the light of the findings from this study.

Chapter 7

Treatment Aspects

INTRODUCTION

The orientation reflected in the foregoing chapter assumes that baby batterers are sick people in need of treatment and help, and that social workers, psychiatrists and other therapists have the knowledge to treat and cure their sickness. Both these assumptions have been questioned by some investigators. Concerning the first point, it has been pointed out that not all incidents of battering have a single set of aetiological factors and consequently while some parents may indeed be ill, others may be quite normal and may merely follow a culturally acceptable child-rearing pattern, perhaps in a somewhat exaggerated manner because of situational stress. Regarding the second assumption, it has been suggested that to the extent that baby batterers are ill, their personality deviations are of a type that is resistant to known methods of treatment, and that psychiatrists and others have only limited success with cases of this type. The following section reviews some of the differing views on treatment aspects.

CONTRASTING VIEWPOINTS

Polansky (1968), an experienced therapist and researcher at the University of Georgia, in reporting to the Joint Commission on Mental Health for Children, questioned the ability of therapists to achieve personality change in battering parents which would assure the welfare of the children. His scepticism led him to view physical abuse of children as 'an area in which social, medical and legal action must be authoritative, intrusive and insistent'. In this report he is also highly critical of the efficacy of casework.

> 'Because of their dedication to the notion of the family or their zeal about "rehabilitation" the formal policies of social agencies in this field are sanguine to the point of being fatuous regarding the potentiality for change in a large proportion of the parents involved. The fact is that most hard-headed observers report little success with the methods of aggressive casework (or unaggressive psychiatry) now being practiced. This is true even when an adequate attempt at treatment is made, something which is possible in only a few areas of the country. The state of the art, in 1968 in the richest nation in history, is poor, even compared with England and Holland.'

Because of these conclusions, Polansky and Polansky (1968) suggested the following seven (abridged) recommendations, 'some of which may seem rather shocking to people unaccustomed to viewing with general detachment the sufferings of children outside their own families'.

(1) 'Wherever there is either clear evidence or even persuasive evidence, of abuse of a child under the age of three, he should be permanently removed from the parental home. Return to the original parental home should be regarded as the rare exception, rather than the hoped-for norm.

(2) Whenever a child is removed from a family because of . . . "battering" . . . the non-guilty parent should be placed on probation and forbidden to remove any other children they have from the possibility of continuous and intensive surveillance by the court of jurisdiction.

(3) The parent found responsible for child battering should be punishable by a substantial term in prison . . . rather than probation. This is because of the known instances in which a parent . . . has still murdered his child even while supposedly on probation.

(4) Children neglected to the point of starvation or actual abandonment by their parents should be promptly removed from the home with the expectation that they will not be returned for a considerable period of time.

(5) The 'failure to thrive' syndrome has been reasonably well established and the findings regarding these cases in which its source lies within the mother's psychological make-up should be made general knowledge among the relevant medical and social agency personnel . . . The law should require that when this is the diagnosis made, the child must be returned for regular check-ups at a suitable . . . clinic. This is to counter the tendency of these mothers to defend against recognizing the problem by 'doctor-shopping'.

(6) The correlation between a low level of child care and large family size is unmistakable, regardless of the cultural or presumed religious backgrounds of those involved . . . Sterilization should be made available to any married person who wants it . . . and . . . should be made available free for those unable to pay.

(7) In view of the evidence before us, it should become a general legal principle that no woman should have to bear a child whom she really does not want . . . This applies to the law regarding abortion, and its availability to low income women, or those unable to manipulate an abortion under the current laws . . . '

Polansky's views concerning the potential effectiveness of therapeutic intervention with respect to reported cases of baby battering differ markedly from those expressed by Steele and Pollock of the University of Colorado School of Medicine. These two psychiatrists are optimistic concerning the potential of psychiatric and social work therapy to modify child rearing patterns of baby batterers, provided that such parents are treated in an accepting, non-punitive manner that meets their own needs for a satisfying and rewarding experience as parents, an experience they have never known in relation to their own parents. Their views are reflected in the following excerpt (Steele and Pollock, 1968).

> 'Our treatment of those who abuse infants has been directed toward improving the basic pattern of child-rearing. It is based upon the hypotheses derived from the study of the psychology of abusing parents in our group. We were able to establish useful contact with all but a few of the sixty families, and of this treated group well over three fourths showed significant improvement. Some changed a great deal, some only moderately, some are still in therapy. We considered it improvement when dangerously severe physical attack of the infant was eliminated and milder physical attack in the form of a disciplinary punishment was either eliminated or reduced to non-injurious minimum. Of equal significance was a reduction in demand upon and criticism of children accompanied by increased recognition of a child as an individual with age appropriate needs and behaviour. Further signs of improvement in the parents were increased abilities to relate to a wider social milieu for pleasurable satisfaction and source of help in time of need rather than looking to their children for such responses.'

It is possible, however, that the success these authors report was dependent upon an externally imposed motivational factor.

> 'Maintenance of contact with us depended upon the admonition from a judge that the parents' probation or the return of their child to them was contingent upon seeing us and a report from us . . . '
>
> (Steele and Pollock, 1968)

Indeed this possibility is exemplified by the observation that a parents' awareness that no confidential material would be released would often lead to a manipulation of therapy, an avoidance of involvement and an 'overtly casual approach to attendance' (Paulson *et al.*, 1971).

Kempe (1971) while accepting that it is 'simply unsafe to have a small child who had been injured returned to parents if one of them is suffering from a major mental illness or is an aggressive psychopath', believes that in the majority of cases 'it is often possible to introduce a therapeutic person while allowing gradual return of the child to the family under continuing treatment'. Indeed, 80 per cent of battered children under his care are returned to their parents within 8 months of initiation of treatment. Only 5 per cent have parental rights permanently terminated, the children then being adopted. It is interesting to contrast Kempe's (1971) views with that expressed almost a decade earlier (Kempe *et al.*, 1962).

> 'In many instances the prompt return of the child to the home is contraindicated because of the threat that additional trauma offers to the childs' health and life . . . the bias should be in favor of the child's safety.'

MOTHERING

Over the last few years Kempe and his colleagues have attempted to treat the deprived parent by 'mothering' (Kempe, 1973), so that emotional dependency on the child and isolation are lessened and feelings of trust are developed. In order to achieve this goal, Kempe and Helfer (1972), have experimented with the use of innovative therapeutic techniques. These include the following.

(1) *Parent Aides* – These are foster grandparents whose job it is to simply cuddle hospitalized children.
(2) *24-Hour Lifeline Services* – These operate on the lines of the Samaritans, and telephone contact with the parents is available 7 days a week.
(3) *Homemaker Services* – These provide battering mothers who are unable to cope with the demands of their small children with support and treatment. 'The Homemaker . . . is one who is willing to work along in a gentle way, by actually helping in the house and with the children, and also providing some of the support'.
(4) *Crisis Nurseries* – These provide 'a place where a child can be safely placed for no other reason than the mothers' relief'.
(5) *Mother's Anonymous* – This is a self help group modelled along the lines of Alcoholics Anonymous and founded in 1970 by a 29-year-old mother known as Jolly K who had almost strangled one of her two children. Kempe and Helfer have described the background of this woman in striking terms.

> 'This woman's educational experiences and preparation for motherhood included approximately 100 foster homes, 32 institutions, rape at age 11 (which she enjoyed, for this was the first time she had actually 'meant anything' to an adult), exotic dancing, prostitution, five years of grade school, a disastrous first and second

> marriage and innumerable negative experiences with men in general. Her background, coupled with her basic innate intelligence, driving personality, seemingly unlimited stamina and fortuitous third marriage, provided the leadership for this new and exciting therapeutic adventure.'

Some of these 'mothering' techniques have also been adopted in the U.K. by the N.S.P.C.C. Battered Child Research Department.

By way of contrast Smith, Hanson and Noble (1974) believe that it is unrealistic to expect baby batterers to take the initiative and avail themselves of such services. Oliver and Cox (1973) in describing the intergenerational aspects of child abuse have shown that baby battering is not diminished by supplying intensive medical and social help to the parents. Oliver *et al.* (1974), have supported Smith, Honigsberger and Smith (1973) and Smith, Hanson and Noble (1974) in their conclusions, and the principle aim of therapy is to ensure the safety of the child and that reliance upon 'mothering' or other methods will be unsuccessful and possibly even dangerous to the child concerned.

> 'The confirmation of the fact that most very cruel parents have been the victims of cruelty can help engender a constructive rather than a punitive attitude. It does not, however, automatically follow that (*a*) such parents would be automatically treated by a "transfusion of mothering" or (*b*) that this is the sole or even the most important aspect of diagnoses when one considers the treatment of a battering parent.'
>
> (Oliver *et al.*, 1974)

GROUP PSYCHOTHERAPY

Following Slavson's introduction of group psychotherapy as a treatment modality in 1955, there has been an increasing recognition and appreciation of this method of therapeutic intervention. Almost every psychiatric disorder has been treated by a group approach with success and failure being well researched and documented. Despite this, there are only isolated reports of group therapy as a method of treating baby batterers.

McFerran (1958), was the first to describe the use of parent groups, but she did not state how many of her families were battering parents. Feinstein, Paul and Esmiol (1964), described the use of group therapy with mothers having infanticidal impulses; however, only one of the mothers had actually battered her child. Zalba (1967), also suggested that group therapy was the treatment of choice but does not provide details of his experience with this technique. Garner (1967), has found that confrontation with baby batterers is effective and Paulson *et al.*

(1971) have strongly advocated a multidisciplinary psychotherapeutic approach to the problem. In their study not only confrontation, but a wide variety of theoretical constructs and therapeutic procedures were used to enhance the personal growth and emotional development of their families in treatment. A control group was not, however, used.

> 'Group psychotherapy as a process of intervention can be successfully applied in the treatment of these individuals and families, who are many times deemed untreatable.'
>
> (Paulson *et al.*, 1971)

Sadoff (1971), in reporting upon the increasing use of compulsory group psychotherapy for criminals, mentioned that there was a lower recidivism rate for criminals having group psychotherapy, than control cases on probation who were given group therapy. His findings, however, caution against predicting future behaviour from a single interview, for the charisma of many of his patient-prisoners swayed evaluator attitudes and led to false predictions.

It thus appears that if psychotherapy as a treatment modality has been used, there is little in the literature showing its applicability and success in the areas working with parents who abuse, batter and maltreat their children.

OTHER METHODS

Galdston (1971) has described the work undertaken by the Parents Center Project for the Study and Prevention of Child Abuse. The Project has treated 23 families with their 42 children over 2 years. The design of the Project is based on two premises.

(1) Child abuse is a disorder of parental ambivalence and this is demonstrated by an unwillingness of the parents to abandon the child or give it up for placement.

(2) The battered child is particularly prone to develop violent behaviour as a character trait because of the abuse he has experienced during his preverbal years.

To overcome these difficulties, the child-care centre offers protective intervention for the child. This allows some distance without separation from his parents. For 8–10 hours, 5 days a week, the child is in the company and under the care of adults other than his parents and 'obtains a different quality of human experience'. The Parents' Group offers its participants some opportunity to share and compare their experience of their children, their marriages and themselves in the hope that they will recognize what difficulties they must call their own rather than attribute to their children.

Galdston (1971), is sceptical regarding the value of foster placements and child-rearing lectures for parents. Because of the success he has achieved with the Parents' Center Project ('none of these 42 children has been physically abused again since they entered the Project'), Galdston has encouraged the creation of other centres. However, he accepts that their prime aim is a holding operation in order to 'buy time'.

Lukianowicz (1971), has had experience of treating 18 battering parents. His efforts have been confined to hospital treatment of the more disturbed parents, and to out-patient individual psychotherapy of the less disturbed parents. These methods brought apparently good results in four mothers and a fair result in five mothers (i.e. 56 per cent of the battering mothers). Lukianowicz (1971) has, however, expressed caution in attributing this success to psychotherapy alone, and is quite pessimistic regarding the successful treatment of battering fathers.

> 'It is only fair to mention that during the course of psychotherapy some of these women were also treated with tranquilizing, and in two cases with anti-depressant drugs. Unfortunately both battering fathers proved to be entirely unco-operative. They refused to come to the clinic and were extremely hostile and abusive to the children's officers, to social workers, and to health visitors, who vainly endeavoured to establish some meaningful relationship with them at their own homes . . . '

Lukianowicz (1971) however, admits that very often, 'the only possible and often unavoidable solution' is to remove the child from the home. A similar view has been expressed by Bennie and Sclare (1969).

> 'On confirmation of child assault, or in cases where this likelihood would appear imminent, steps must be taken to separate child from parent until the crisis has passed.'

Ounsted and his colleagues at the Park Hospital for Children, Oxford, believe that 'bonding failure', is an important underlying factor in the psychopathology of baby batterers. Because of this they have encouraged the development of an 'open relationship' that entails 'removing both physically and emotionally all the constraints which have held the family closed' (Ounsted, Oppenheimer and Lindsay, 1974). Ounsted has described his experience of treating two series of patients. One group consisted of approximately 50 battering families and another group comprised 24 mothers who were selected for treatment because of fears that they might injure their babies. Ounsted found that serious mental illness, psychopathy and inadequate personalities were present in the majority of cases but fails to provide precise statistics for the prevalence of these disorders. 'We do not think statistical treatment of such complex data is at present desirable'. He has described the regime used at the Park Hospital, in the following way.

> 'We place the families in a highly regressed state. They are fed, housed, cared for as though they were infants. It might seem a paradox that in this situation they can change and mature. But consider how a caterpillar changes into a butterfly —the regression of pupation is essential. Thus we see the simultaneous occurrence of psychodynamic dissolution and psychodynamic developmental advance, not as a paradox but rather . . . a resolution by the coming together of opposites.'

In describing the outcome of treatment Ounsted and his colleagues have warned against generalizing from selected groups. However, they found that 33.3 per cent were untreatable in the sense that permanent removal of the child under a Care Order was required, the same figure that Smith, Honigsberger and Smith (1973) found. Among the remainder a notable improvement in the intra-familial dynamics with no relapse occurring among fully treated families took place. However 'no statistics of outcome would be meaningful since both our ideas and our practice are in a state of evolution'.

Isaacs (1972), has emphasized the importance of psychiatric assessment on the parents concerned, but in contrast to Ounsted, Oppenheimer and Lindsay (1974), and others (Steele and Pollock, 1968; Galdston, 1971), she regards interpretative psychotherapy as rarely being required. Isaacs recommends instead, that reliance be placed upon 'benign supervision' by some person 'trained or untrained . . . who can, without blaming or condoning convey an understanding of the need to keep the child safe and well'.

By way of contrast several authors (Smith, 1972; Oliver *et al.*, 1974; Howells, 1974) have criticized current approaches to the battered baby problem. In his interesting book *'Remember Maria'*, Howells (1974) reveals the misconceptions that lie behind present practices. His particular attack is upon the reluctance of social workers and others to separate the child from its mother.

> 'This misconception about the mother–child bond is strongly held and denies the evident pain that it sometimes causes to the child. It is reminiscent of the Inquisition, where the greatest pain, indignity, degradation, violence, misuse of justice and death were still justified by a wrongfully held belief.'

Howells forcefully expresses the opinion that society's subscription to 'wrong ideas' was responsible for the death of Maria Colwell. He has also remarked that the very services created to help battered children add to the risks these children face.

Oliver *et al.* (1974) believe that because the suffering of these young children has been so intense and the consequences of parental cruelty so devastating, that arguments in favour of more efficient methods of surveillance and control 'must outweigh the (mainly theoretical) objections'.

Kempe (1973), in concluding his report to the United States Senate has drawn an interesting parallel between inadequate parenting and marital breakdown.

> 'Society has worked out a way to manage failure in marriage; it is called divorce. We should be prepared to accept failures in totally unregulated, random parenthood by permitting, without social stigma, either voluntary or involuntary termination of parental rights for children from those parents who cannot, for one reason or another, give them the minimal physical and emotional support they deserve.'

CUSTODIAL TREATMENTS

Walker (1968) in his excellent review of the legal aspects of infanticide has pointed out that 'what most judges seem to have found objectionable was the necessity of pronouncing the death penalty on the mothers who were convicted of murder'. It was argued that such women must be insane, and as a result the Infanticide Act, 1938 was passed. This resulted in a decreasingly punitive attitude by the courts towards such a crime and a declining percentage of women who were being imprisoned for it. This effect contrasts strikingly, with Hood's statement (quoted in Walker and McCabe, 1973), to the Capital Punishment Commission nearly a century earlier that 'it was advisable to detain infanticidal women until they had passed child bearing age'.

Such a remarkable shift in sentencing pattern must of course be viewed against a perspective in which there has been a general shrinking in the use of imprisonment. Indeed 'the virtual abandonment of prison sentences as a means of dealing with crime involving the taking of human life is one of the most striking developments in the history of our sentencing policy' (Walker, 1968). It is now exceptional for a woman to be imprisoned for infanticide; disposal usually rests with probation with or without a condition of psychiatric treatment (Walker, 1968; d'Orban, 1974).

The effectiveness of such techniques in treating such mothers has never been accurately assessed. However, Bluglass (1974), a forensic psychiatrist, has found probation with a condition of psychiatric treatment a useful alternative to imprisonment. His treatment is eclectically orientated. Scott (1973), commenting on a group of fathers who killed their young children, suggests that a small proportion can be handled as at present without any custodial sentence and is optimistic that as knowledge and facilities for treatment improve then this proportion can certainly be increased. Other aspects of custodial treatments as they applied to this study will be described later.

CONCLUSION

This review has shown that there is at present no consensus of opinion about the management of cases in which a child has been injured by his parents. Treatment is based on broad principles, the social worker being in the key position to intervene in this multidisciplinary problem. There seems to be a strong need for systematic research on such families and a designing of reliable measures that will assess those families at risk. This, of course, encroaches upon prevention of baby battering.

Though very little has been written about preventive aspects, several authors (Kempe, 1973; Court, 1973; Ounsted, Oppenheimer and Lindsay, 1974) believe that the goal that should be reached is the ascertainment of families at risk during the antenatal stage. Indeed, Kempe (1973) is optimistic that this can be achieved.

> 'A number of predictive studies are currently underway and there is reason to believe that it will be possible to identify parents at risk in the pre-natal period, during the first hour of mother/child interaction, and in the early post-natal period. Once a risk family is identified, it is possible to begin active intervention through the utilization of well accepted supportive health contacts such as visiting nurses, frequent well-baby visits, phone calls from a sympathetic physician and mobilization of family resources and friends.'

Admirable though this aim is our current knowledge of predictive studies remains at the developmental stage (Schneider, Helfer and Pollock, 1972). Furthermore, it has already been established that active intervention does not always result in rehabilitation of the family. Evidence from this study will later show that prevention of re-battering is but a crude index of successful treatment, and that many battered children are at risk of social maldevelopment and death.

Chapter 8

Court Procedure

INTRODUCTION

Recent growing awareness of tragic instances of battered baby cases in professional literature and the daily press have prompted an outraged public to demand that 'something be done'. Following the Kempe *et al.* (1962) report, many states in America responded with constructive measures that were aimed at providing greater protection for children. Sometimes however the pressure has been for additional punitive laws, with little attention made to the broader legal framework required for effective child-care protection.

Raising children has been the concern of parents and not of government. The law has therefore given parents the custody of children and has relied upon parental love to provide the care and protection a child requires. It is not surprising therefore to note that baby battering takes place in a setting which the legal system has arranged. The law has however provided for intervention by society when parental care is dangerously faulty or insufficient.

Two separate types of proceedings can result from the investigation of the alleged non-accidental injury to children.

(1) Criminal proceedings against one or both parents or guardians in the adult courts.

(2) Care proceedings in respect of the child in the juvenile courts.

Each court has a different jurisdiction and a different basis for trial and disposal. The following section broadly examines the legal framework in which the battered child is dealt with in the United Kingdom and discusses some of the legal issues involved.

CRIMINAL PROCEEDINGS

Grounds for legal action may result in either civil or criminal proceedings and sometimes both. The criminal case is brought in the adult court since the point at issue is whether or not the adult has rendered himself liable to be dealt with under the criminal law. The case is usually brought under the Children and Young Persons Act, 1933, section 1, on the grounds of cruelty of a specified kind, and is usually completed in the magistrates' court (Graham-Hall, 1975). In a very few cases and where there is a definite wound the charge is brought under the Offences Against the Person Act, 1861, section 18, and this must be heard in the higher court. In either event the prosecution must, if it is to succeed, have evidence which pins the responsibility on to one or more specified individuals. The sentencing powers of the court include imprisonment.

Low (1971) has discussed at length the courses open to the prosecution when dealing with these cases. These include: murder, attempted murder, infanticide, manslaughter, various offences under sections 18 and 20 of the Offences Against the Person Act, 1861, assault occasioning actual bodily harm and statutory offences of cruelty and neglect. For the defence he considers only three courses open; diminished responsibility, provocation and accident.

> 'The criminal law is quite adequate for any purpose it may serve in this area without more being created, a fact which public opinion, roused by newspaper reports of sensational cases, sometimes tends to forget in its enthusiasm for new but unnecessary punitive legislation.'
>
> (Low, 1971)

The criminal procedure however is not in practice quite as useful as might at first sight be expected (Cavenagh, 1974). Firstly, it may be impossible to secure a conviction because there are often no witnesses to the acts alleged and the accused persons refuse to incriminate themselves. For this reason some police feel that the ends of justice are likely to be defeated if they, as expert interrogators of suspects in criminal cases, are not brought on to the scene until after questioning by doctors and/or social workers has alerted the suspect to possible lines of defence (Robinson, 1973; Mounsey, 1975). Secondly, if the defence is 'accident', it may be impossible to prove the '*mens rea*' required for conviction. Thirdly, the trend of social policy and social work training has been to keep the family together at all costs, for it is argued that offending parents and their victims can only be rehabilitated *in situ* and as part of family education (Howells, 1974).

The law however is geared to imposing penal sanctions upon an offending individual but has the power to make a probation order. This provides a situation in which it is sometimes possible for reform to take place. The court, however, has no power to make an order relating to the battered child. Since 1969 it has had no power to order that such a child be brought before the juvenile court, because it was thought that the possibility of bringing care proceedings will have been considered already (Cavenagh, 1974). There is thus no statutory machinery by which the court can draw the attention of the social services to the situation. It may of course do so informally and it is the practice of the police to notify the Social Services departments of such cases. However 'an alarming lack of liaison' often occurs between all these agencies (Graham-Hall, 1975).

CARE PROCEEDINGS

The case in the juvenile court is under its civil jurisdiction and the point at issue is the quality of care being received by the child and likely to be received in the future (Goodman, 1974). Proceedings are brought under the Children and Young Persons Act, 1969, section 1(2), on the grounds that:

(*a*) 'The proper development of the child is being avoidably prevented or neglected or his health is being avoidably impaired or neglected or he is being ill treated, and also

(*b*) that he is in need of care or control which he is unlikely to receive unless the court makes an order.'

Care proceedings may be brought by a local authority, the police or the N.S.P.C.C. In most instances they are brought by one of the first two (Cavenagh, 1974). The burden of proof required is not, as in a criminal case, such as places the matter beyond a reasonable doubt, but it is the lower civil standard of proof which enables issues to be decided upon the balance of probabilities (Cavenagh, 1967). Conviction in the adult court can shorten and simplify proceedings in the juvenile court for it provides part of the evidence required. In practice if juvenile court proceedings are contemplated, these are held back pending the outcome in the adult court. The parent in the meantime is usually on bail, and the child is in the care of the social services department, on an interim order, or in hospital. No final assessment of the child's needs and no definite plans for his future can be made, nor can case-work proceed until it is known whether the parent is going to be removed from the scene by a prison sentence. Prolonged delay, may of course, increase the emotional side of whatever has already been suffered by the child.

If the parent is acquitted in the adult court this does not necessarily mean that the juvenile court case will fail. The essential matters to be proved in the juvenile court are the facts of the child's situation and not necessarily who is responsible for causing it. Thus the allegations may be proved without the court necessarily being certain as to whether it was the father, the mother, or any other culprit. A case may also be proved to the courts' satisfaction even though it has not shown that the damage was non-accidental, in the sense of being intended, or due to conscious recklessness; for the point at issue is the child's actual situation now and probable situation in the future, not the culpability *per se* of whoever did the damage. In practice this allows a successful case to be brought and the child to be protected, even though the baby batterer cannot be brought to justice through lack of evidence (Goodman, 1973).

TYPES OF ORDER

Before any case comes to court whether as a criminal charge against an adult and/or a care or control case of the child, the police or other authorized prosecuting authority exercises a discretion whether to bring proceedings. When they have ascertained all the relevant facts they decide what action is appropriate. In exercising this discretion, the seriousness of the allegations, the likelihood of recurrence, the probability of the case being prosecuted are all considered.

The grounds of complaint are so defined in the Children and Young Persons Act, 1969, however, that it is difficult to envisage a complaint being brought at all. Cavenagh (1974) has criticized the social services departments for not stating clearly, on the basis of their examination of the situation and their expertise in child welfare, what order is in their view required to ensure that the child obtains the care he needs. This does not mean that the court in deciding upon the order will simply rubber-stamp the social services department's view. If arrangements for care have not been made on a voluntary basis and it has been thought necessary to bring the child before the court, it may be argued that a state of conflict exists or is regarded as more than a possibility. There exist, therefore, two points of view, namely as to whether an order, and if so what order, should be made. In practice the choice is almost always between a supervision order, which does not give the local authority power to remove the child and a care order which does.

Care orders may be made because supervision alone may be sparse and inadequate in picking up and acting promptly upon indications of present and impending danger. In some cases the court or the social services department itself may wish the latter to have in reserve, power to remove a child at a moment's notice at any time, without arguments or effective opposition, on even the suspicion of danger if they feel this to be necessary. Care orders are not, however, removal orders, although a court making a care order usually assumes that the child will be removed at once. A care order simply confers powers on the local authority which the latter may or may not exercise at its own discretion and entirely on its own responsibility.

Smith and Hanson (1974), have criticized the misuse of this responsibility by local authorities. Cavenagh (1974) has succinctly stated the problem.

> 'Expertise and decision making in the local authority is . . . crucial in ensuring that decisions are not taken on the basis of mere suppositions which have not been put in issue before the court.'

CRITICISM OF THE CURRENT JURISDICTION

Several authors (Fetherstone, 1972; Smith and Noble, 1973; Goodman and Power, 1973; Cavenagh 1974; Goodman, 1974; Graham-Hall, 1975) have criticized certain aspects of the present legal situation.

Fetherstone (1972) has argued that the objectives of the Children and Young Persons Act, 1969, have been 'frustrated by its own machinery' and feels that the Children and Young Persons Act, 1933, maintained a better balance between the conflicting interests which exist in these cases. He suggests that the second requirement of the 1969 Act has proved the stumbling block.

> 'If the parent even freely acknowledges his fault but convinces the court that it was a single lapse which will not recur the court has no choice but to dismiss the case . . . Already a number of such cases have produced tragic results of second and very much more severe sets of injuries.'

Smith and Noble (1973) have pointed out that in contrast to adult courts the juvenile courts have no power to require the parents to submit themselves to psychiatric examination in order to help the court decide upon the appropriate order. Reliance instead is placed upon a social enquiry report. Cavenagh (1974) has supported Smith and Noble's (1973) recommendation for psychiatric reports, but pointed out that some parents can at present be 'blackmailed into doing this'.

Goodman and Power (1973) have shown that London Boroughs vary in their practice of allowing legal representation for the child and that juvenile courts differ markedly in the types of orders they issue. In 16.6 per cent of their cases the parents were prosecuted, but there was marked variation between the Boroughs in initiating and successfully completing a prosecution.

Graham-Hall (1975) has pointed out other difficulties that may arise on disposal. The care or supervision order in the Magistrates Court or Crown Court is made in the form of a probation order. Whichever type of supervision order is in existence the court which made it does not have any power unless the supervisor takes the case back to it. In practice, the juvenile court may issue a care order and yet the child can be returned to the parents with no consultation made by the social services department either with the court, the paediatrician or any other interested agency (Goodman, 1974). Graham-Hall has suggested that one solution to this problem would be to make a condition of medical supervision of the child part of the court order, on the same lines that it is a prerequisite of a probation order that the adult agrees to the terms of the order. This would mean that the parents would be required to take the child at regular intervals to a named medical practitioner for check-ups.

Cavenagh (1974) has suggested that it is probably unwise even for unopposed applications for revocation of care orders to be heard in the absence of the child concerned. Perhaps other persons, such as the foster parents who have been immediately concerned in his care, should be notified and have a right to appear and be heard. Certainly this suggestion seems sound and might even prevent tragedies similar to the Maria Colwell case (Howells, 1974).

Another criticism has been not so much in the powers of adult or juvenile courts, as in the provision of the social services. Cavenagh (1974) has exemplified this point.

> 'One of the most difficult types of case is one in which there has been a short history of several accidental injuries at different times in the first six–nine months of life, from which the child has made an excellent recovery and is now before the court on a further allegation of injury, which is proved. In a recent case the parents appeared as a capable and loving 20 year old mother with a husband of similar age but completely unused to handling any small animal. It was he who had "accidentally" caused a further fracture. Though extraordinarily clumsy he appeared well intentioned and loving . . . Should the child now be taken into care with the risk of emotional damage, since 24-hour minute-by-minute supervision is otherwise impossible? In cases of this kind could there not be provision for training for fathers which courts could require to be undertaken as an alternative to prison or otherwise?'

Smith and Noble (1973) have pointed out that a case may be lost because a doctor may be prevented by the Clerk or the parents' lawyer from giving evidence which he regards as highly significant to the general picture. The writer has been criticized when giving evidence at the juvenile court on the grounds that the term 'battered baby' is unknown to the law.

Courts also vary in their practice as to what they regard as admissable evidence (Goodman, 1973). Expert witnesses are often perplexed by questions based upon the concepts of 'certainty' and courts vary in their practice of explaining the procedure beforehand. Social workers may never have been in court before, and yet the practice of having a staff member who can act as a court officer and who is familiar with court procedure and its pitfalls, varies throughout the United Kingdom (Cavenagh, 1974).

The Criminal Law Revision Committee is presently studying some of these points (Tunbridge Wells Study Group, 1973) but has not as yet issued a statement pertaining to the legal procedures in battered baby cases. Their deliberations are awaited with interest.

LESSONS LEARNED FROM THE MARIA COLWELL REPORT

Maria Colwell was born on March 25, 1965. For the first 6 years of her life she was fostered by her aunt and uncle, and for most of that time she was in the care of the East Sussex County Council by order of the Hove Juvenile Court. In November, 1971, her mother applied to the court for the revocation of the care order and the return of her child. The county council did not oppose the application, and the court granted it. Maria was taken home to her mother and stepfather where, by another order of the court, the county council remained responsible for her supervision. Fourteen months later, a few weeks before her eighth birthday, she died of multiple injuries received at the hands of her stepfather Mr. William Kepple, who was found guilty of murder, a finding of manslaughter being substituted by the Court of Appeal. Her death was the culmination of months of ill-treatment.

A committee of three, under the chairmanship of Mr. T. G. Field-Fisher, QC, was set up to find out what it was that had gone wrong with the public arrangement for looking after children in need of care and protection. Apart from the sweeping observation that 'it is upon society as a whole that the ultimate blame must rest', the report (Department of Health and Social Security, 1974) provides a most valuable picture of the social services in action and makes a fair apportionment of responsibility.

The members of the committee were not unanimous, but their differences were more of emphasis than otherwise. Miss Olive Stevenson,

Reader in Social Administration at Oxford, was more lenient in her comments on particular social workers engaged in the case and more conscious of the difficulties of their task. All were agreed, however, that individual mistakes and errors of judgement were made – though the significance of them is much more evident in hindsight than it could have been at the time – and all were agreed that primarily the trouble was a failure of the system: the failure of professionals and caseworkers in a multiplicity of agencies to compare notes with one another, or even to be aware of one anothers' activity in the same case and the failure of administrators to devise and maintain a system which has safeguards against the consequences of only-to-be-expected human error.

The report concentrates, in particular, on the almost total lack of information about William Kepple. That deficiency highlights the difficulty which social workers appear to be having in gaining knowledge about all the members of a family. When a foster child was badly assaulted some years ago in Dorset (also the subject of official injury), the culprit was another foster-child living in the same home. Certainly, husbands and fathers are often shadowy figures in the pictures of family life which social workers construct. Where step-parents are concerned, the report rightly maintains that especial care must be taken to include them.

Other vital matters emerge about how information, once obtained, is interpreted. In this case, much depended on how Maria's reactions to the occasional visits to her mother were understood. The local authority social worker told the inquiry that she 'had to make an intelligent guess'. The sometimes turbulent scenes preceding the visits, and the occasions when she ran away, were not considered to be abnormal in such a situation. The danger, of course, is that social workers who are constantly exposed to stressful circumstances may come to redefine their conceptions of normality and the meaning of dramatic behaviour. The main report concludes that the stress Maria showed when trial visits to her mother were arranged was extraordinary, and was a measure of her reluctance.

The report repeatedly reminds us about the problems of communicating with children in distress. When and how should they be seen alone? How far should we rely on what they tell us, and how far depend on what we see or, indeed, touch? Only a teacher seems ever to have held Maria and felt how thin and light she was. In particular, how are we to interpret what a child tells us when we believe her to be caught in a web of mixed and tormenting loyalties?

It appears from the report that three mistakes neutralized any action to remove Maria. One was the N.S.P.C.C. Inspector's wrong conclusions about the cause of the injuries. The second was the reliance placed on that conclusion by the social worker with responsibility for the supervision. The last was a failure to obtain, by any means, a medical opinion. By contrast, the neighbours conviction was not accorded enough weight. The decision not to treat the situation as grave, undoubtedly affected attitudes to the later events. That must surely be the reason why further disturbing evidence, which emerged in the next few days, did not cause change of mind or an intensification of the supervision.

All might not have been lost if the subsequent signs of maltreatment had been available to one or other of the social workers who had inquired into the first complaint. In fact, from this point on, the number of interested agencies and individuals proliferated, and information grew more dispersed and unco-ordinated: these were the police, the school, the educational welfare officers, the health visitor, the general practitioner and the housing department.

Three main factors aggravated the disorganization of information and collapse of communication. First, the local authority social worker assumed that supervision was being carried out by the N.S.P.C.C., and effectively withdrew for 6 months. It is noteworthy that cases of cruelty to children are some of the most likely to create an ambiguous involvement of statutory and voluntary organizations. Second, two local authorities were sharing responsibility. The overlap of responsibility bears a sad resemblance to the O'Neill case in the 1940s (in that case, it was the foster-parent who killed a child) (*see* the Report by Sir Walter Monckton, 1945). The wisdom of such arrangements may need to be rethought. Third, at least four 'examinations' of Maria did take place at some point. After a further complaint to the N.S.P.C.C., their inspector and the local authority social worker both saw Maria stripped. When this revealed no signs of bruising, they were relieved and one imagines, confirmed in their first judgement.

Evidently there is no one simple organizational reform, like the administrative integration of all welfare functions, which is going to prevent these kinds of failure. The points of contact between public servants and private citizens, even those who do not present any kind of 'problem' to authority, are by now so many and various that administrative partitions are unavoidable. If relevant information is to be better shared it will have to be by means of a greater flow of paper or greater altertness among field workers to pass on and look out for information which might be to the point.

There is however one point at which the need for a change in procedure stands out very clearly from this report. The turning point in the outward drama of Maria Colwell's life was the hearing before the Hove

Juvenile Court in November 1971 when the care order was discharged permitting Maria's mother to regain custody of her. The application went through more or less on the nod, the magistrates having before them the social worker's report and hearing brief evidence from Maria's mother. As the report of the inquiry points out, once the county council had decided (for reasons which must now be judged to be wrong, but which were far from careless or perverse) not to oppose a course which led to Maria's removal from her foster-parents and restoration to her mother and stepfather, there was no examination before the courts of the arguments for not allowing this to happen. Yet the arguments for and against, in the light of the evidence considered by the county council, were fairly evenly matched – and had it been someone's duty to argue the case against, further evidence would certainly have been brought forth.

The committee of inquiry recommended that in this type of situation a second opinion of an independent social worker should always be available to the court – 'the local authority are, after all, an actual party to the proceedings'. Mrs Barbara Castle, the Secretary of State, in her comments on the report, adds that she is considering for possible inclusion in a Children's Bill the provision that in certain court proceedings the child's interests should be protected by separate legal representation.These improvements can now be seen to be necessary.

THE CHILDREN BILL

At the time of writing, the House of Lords have completed their debate on The Children Bill, which completed its report stage on March 6.

The Bill, which largely follows the lines of the report of the Houghton Committee on adoption, attempts a general reformulation of the law on adoption, guardianship, and children in care. It proposes a new professional adoption service to deal with the 24 000 cases a year now coming forward. A new 'relinquishment' procedure is introduced to cut short the period of uncertainty which adoptive parents now face. A new status, midway between adoption and fostering, is created, which the Bill calls 'custodianship' – a term which has been criticized on the grounds that it carries a ring of the prison gate about it. The powers of local authorities over children in care are substantially extended. Naturally there was overwhelming concern in the Lords to make sure that such a comprehensive reform of the law would be watertight enough to prevent children from meeting the same fate as Maria Colwell. Another powerful constraint has also arisen. In the past few years there have been measures, of which the 1969 Children and Young Persons Act and the 1970 Chronically Sick and Disabled Persons Act are the most conspicuous, whose good intentions have failed because they imposed demands on money and manpower which could not be met. Indeed, in the case of the Children and Young Persons Act, the subsequent disillusionment has been such that the motives behind the reform have to some extent become discredited.

Local authorities are already deeply apprehensive about the demands which the reforming intentions of The Children Bill may make on them. Dr. David Owen, Minister of State for Health, who first introduced this measure in a different form as a private member's Bill in 1973, and will now take it through the Commons, has been meeting local-government organizations to assure them that their difficulties are appreciated and that the introduction of the Bill's provisions will be very carefully phased with their problems in mind. But their fears are far from allayed. Lady Young, from the Conservative front bench, drew attention on February 4 to the views of directors of social services, who believed that the impact on local authorities had been very seriously underestimated by the Government. Indeed nowhere did the present services meet the standard which the new Bill seeks to set.

Economic constraints were also mustered against the most radical critics of the Bill – those who argued that people who wanted to help vulnerable children ought to start by improving standards of housing and by trying to eradicate poverty: the implementation of the Finer Report on one-parent families was several times cited as an essential ingredient in this strategy.

There were other debates, of course, which turned more on philosophical than on financial considerations. Had the Bill gone far enough in seeing that the welfare of the child was given its proper weight? The Lords thought not, passing an amendment to make the child's welfare the primary consideration in decisions on adoption by courts and adoption agencies – though another amendment stipulating that the child's welfare must be 'paramount' when decisions were made on children in care was not pressed. Much of this ground will be covered again in the Commons, when once more the balance between the dictates of compassion and those of available resources seems likely to dominate the debate.

Chapter 9

Medical Reporting of Child Abuse: The American Experience

PATTERNS OF REPORTING

Guidelines for legislation to regulate the reporting of child abuse developed by the U.S. Children's Bureau (*The Abused Child*, 1963), and the American Humane Association (1963), have already been mentioned. It has been noted that these guidelines differed in their recommendations concerning the official agency to whom reports should be made. The Children's Bureau recommended that reports be made to the police, since police authorities function in every community 24 hours a day. The Humane Association recommended public or private protective agencies as recipients of the reports, since these agencies were thought to be better qualified than the police in dealing with battered baby cases in a protective non-punitive and therapeutic manner. Both these guidelines failed to suggest specifically that fatal incidents be reported and that medical examiners or coroners be required to report fatalities they suspected were the result of physical abuse. This oversight was carried over into all laws that were eventually enacted on the basis of the guidelines with the exception of the laws passed by Arkansas, Hawaii and Oregon (Gil, 1970).

Controversy immediately arose after the Children's Bureau published its legislative guidelines. The American Medical Association thought that the guidelines discriminated against physicians singling them out as the only professional group responsible for reporting and was concerned that parents would avoid bringing their children for medical care following an injury for fear of being suspected and reported (*Journal of the American Medical Association* 1964). The American Medical Association also suggested that, in addition to physicians, school personnel, social workers and nurses should be required to report, since physicians tended to be the last professional group to see injured children. These people were also thought to be more effective in bringing about early protective intervention. The American Medical Association subsequently also developed its own legislative proposal which left reporting to the discretion of physicians, nurses, teachers and social workers, rather than making it mandatory. The recipients of the reports in the American Medical Association's proposal were child welfare agencies or the police.

In 1965, the Council of State Governments published its model reporting law which was a compromise between the Children's Bureau and the American Humane Association guidelines (Gil, 1970). Finally, in 1966 the Committee on the Infant and Pre-School Child of the American Academy of Pediatrics (Chairman: Samuel Karelitz) published its recommendations concerning the reporting of child abuse incidents (American Academy of Pediatrics, 1966). In contrast to the American Medical Association's recommendations the Academy favoured mandatory reporting by physicians to child welfare or police authorities. It also recommended the inclusion of a mandatory service clause in the law, and the establishment of central registries of reported incidents at the state level, with provisions for elimination of names of persons included in the registry for insufficient reasons. All the guidelines and legislative proposals recommended the granting of immunity from civil and criminal liability to persons making reports in good faith.

By the middle of 1967 all states in America had enacted laws concerning the reporting of baby battering. Reporting is discretional in six states – Alaska, Missouri, New Mexico, North Carolina, Texas and Washington – but mandatory in all other states. There are differences in the 52 laws concerning the age of a child up to which injuries are reportable, the professional groups required to report, the official agencies to whom reports are to be made, the responsibilities and rights of persons making reports and of the official recipients of reports, the establishment of central registries and penalties for failing to report under the law (Paulsen, 1968). These differences reflect not only different interests in the states, but also the conflicting positions of the various groups who developed guidelines. Several comparative summaries of the various American laws have been published since 1964 (American Humane Association, 1964, 1966; McCoid, 1965; Paulsen, 1966, 1967; Children's Bureau, 1966; Paulsen, Parker and Adelman, 1966).

PROBLEMS OF REPORTING

Soon after the laws were enacted it became clear that several problems limited the effectiveness of reporting as a measure toward prevention, treatment and control. Firstly, many physicians, especially those in private practice, continued to be either unaware of the provisions of the law, or though aware, hesitant to co-operate in implementing its provisions. As a result reporting was erratic and tended to reflect different levels of interest and co-operation on the part of local medical practitioners and others, rather than the real incidence of child abuse (Gil, 1970).

Silver, Barton and Dublin (1967) concluded on the basis of a survey of 450 physicians (half of whom responded), that 'physicians are not sufficiently aware of the battered child syndrome or of community procedures for the management of cases of child abuse'. One in five physicians reported rarely or never considering child abuse when seeing an injured child, one in six said they had failed to consider child abuse in a case that might have been child abuse and more than half the physicians said they did not know the correct procedure to follow in their community. Nearly one quarter of all the physicians stated that he would not report a case of suspected battered child syndrome even if he were protected against legal action by the parents; the physicians main concern being the evidence would not stand up in a court proceeding.

> 'Other considerations that appear to inhibit the physician from reporting his suspicion of child abuse include difficulty on the part of the physician in accepting the reality of wilful child abuse . . . and confusion over the meaning and scope of many basic terms describing child neglect and abuse.'
> (Silver, Barton and Dublin, 1967)

A second and perhaps even more serious problem also became apparent following the reporting of battered child incidents. This concerned the inadequacy of child welfare services in many communities throughout the U.S.A. Because of lack of adequate services for dealing constructively with the battered child and his family reporting was turned into a futile formality. Paulsen (1966) has succinctly summarized the situation based on his experience of legally protecting the battered child.

> 'Reporting is, of course, not enough. After a report is made something has to happen. A multidisciplinary network of protection needs to be developed in each community to implement the good intention of the law. If child protective services are not available, reporters will no longer report. The promise of case finding legislation such as reporting laws, is that when a case is found, something is done about it. The legislators, which require reporting but do not provide the means for further protective action delude themselves and neglect children.'

A third problem arose over 'due process' of law (Gil, 1970). Kimberley Cheney of the School of Law at Yale University has pointed out that because the primary purpose of reporting legislation is the protection of the safety of children, then efforts to assure this safety may at times infringe upon the constitutional rights of parents and even of the children themselves. He has commented on various aspects of this complicated issue.

> 'The best way to assure both that due process of law is observed and that the values on which decisions are made are clearly stated is by providing parents with counsel if they cannot do so themselves. . . Lawyers could help force those persons concerned with child (abuse and) neglect to grapple with the basic social and legal questions involved. Thus, a protective statute should make provision for counsel at the time of the court review, if requested, and clients should be informed of the right on the initial contact.'
>
> (Cheney, 1966)

Co-operation between medical, welfare and legal authorities, and efforts to improve mutual understanding of the different responsibilities assigned to them by society, is viewed by Cheney (1966) as the best chance for minimizing the inherent conflict between on the one hand, an emphasis on the child's safety and on the other, an emphasis on due process and constitutional rights for the parent.

A final set of problems concerns the appropriateness of legal and administrative provisions of specific laws for constructive, protective intervention, and the feasibility of such intervention. Many psychiatrists and social workers dislike reporting to law enforcement agencies since these agencies may symbolize a punitive rather than a helpful attitude by the community toward the parent (Gil, 1970).

Silver (1968) feels that the best approach is a social service approach, in which the major goals are to protect the child and to assist the family in making use of whatever community facilities it may need.

> 'After evaluating the parent or parents, appropriate action can be initiated. Some parents may need social or psychiatric help, some parents may need hospitalization, other parents may need criminal court action. Penalizing the parent or placing the parent in jail does not help the problem; in fact in many cases it may complicate the problem by depriving the family of the wage earner or by removing the mother, thus creating the need for a variety of community services . . . By offering help and not prosecution, the parents will be more available to look at the family difficulties and to accept community assistance in coping with the difficulties.'

Simons and Downs (1968) have concisely summarized the accomplishments of reporting legislation in New York City.

> 'If the intent of legislating child abuse reporting was to abet the movement to broaden availability and the scope of protective and preventive services for children, then legislation has been successful . . . However, if the principal intent of the law was to increase case finding substantially it seems doubtful that this goal has been achieved.'

Certainly the passage of these laws appeased public concern; 'like the air raid siren these laws, when cases are reported, call attention to a dangerous situation', (de Francis, 1972). In the long term, however, solutions to the problem of baby battering call for an enlightened population willing to identify the children and families involved and an acceptance of responsibilities implied in the social concepts of the law. Should this utopia be achieved, the need for legislation might well disappear.

REPORTING IN BRITAIN

The failure of reporting in the United States and the problems that it has produced should not deter authorities from seriously considering statutory reporting in the United Kingdom. Bevan (1975), a member of the Tunbridge Wells Study Group, raised five questions relevant to this issue.

(1) Should there be a legal duty to report?
(2) What should be the scope of reporting?
(3) On whom would the duty fall to report?
(4) How may this duty be discharged?
(5) What would be the object of reporting?

Many members of the Study Group favoured mandatory reporting, but many opposed it. Ingram (1973) foresaw no support for new legislation that introduced mandatory reporting procedures; this is also the present view of the D.H.S.S. (Owen, 1974). The Study Group concluded that more information would be required before a sound decision could be reached and proposed that a working party should be established that would collect information on reporting, registering and notification in the United Kingdom. This working party would also report on the 'advantages, difficulties and disadvantages' of such schemes. The outcome of this resolution is awaited with interest.

CONCLUSION

The foregoing review of the work of researchers and professionals in the field suggests that some progress has been achieved during the past decade towards a better understanding of baby battering and its aetiology and also in society's ability to deal with the problem. At the same time, few questions concerning the psychiatric and social aspects and the most appropriate response to it have been answered satisfactorily. Disagreement among professionals continues to exist with regard to nearly every aspect of the battered child phenomenon – its scope, its nature and measures for dealing with it.

PART II

ONE HUNDRED AND THIRTY-FOUR BATTERED CHILDREN AND THEIR PARENTS: A CONTROLLED STUDY

Chapter 10

Outline of the Study

PURPOSE OF THE STUDY

The previous chapters have shown that although generalizations describing the characteristic features of parents who batter babies have recently become prominent, there is a scarcity of controlled studies. Recent observations have suggested that battering parents are not confined to any particular personality type, intelligence level or social class (Steele and Pollock, 1968) and that 'child abuse is psychodynamically-related and has nothing to do with race, colour, sex, creed, income, education or anything else' (Kempe, 1969). By way of contrast other authors have noted that battering parents are young (Gil, 1968*b*) and from the lower social classes (Young, 1964; Skinner and Castle, 1969). Mental illness and subnormality have been observed by several authors (Woolley and Evans, 1955; Birrell and Birrell, 1968; Lukianowicz, 1971). In addition Gibbens and Walker (1956) mention that criminality and alcoholism are often found. In contrast other authors believe that those who injure their children are not aggressive criminals but relatively normal persons who are exposed to unusual and excessive stress (Helfer and Kempe, 1968). The view has also been put forward that psychopathy is not a significant finding (Steele and Pollock, 1968). Despite this it has been shown that a high proportion of baby batterers have a history of blackouts or fits (Gibbens and Walker, 1956).

Despite clinical descriptions of battered children (Adelson, 1961; Weston, 1968; Gregg and Elmer, 1969; Harcourt and Hopkins, 1971; Mushin, 1971) there has been no previous comprehensive and controlled study which has included both medical and psychological assessments.

Because the correct diagnosis is often missed and because doctors are still unsuspecting (Lancet, 1971), this study reports birth abnormalities, age, sex, types and degree of injury and their sequelae in 134 battered children. Other factors thought to be important in precipitating a battering incident are also described.

A knowledge of parental characteristics seemed to the author to be of prime importance in the management of the battered baby syndrome. Because previous studies have led to conflicting conclusions it was decided also to undertake a controlled investigation of their parents. This study compares, age, psychiatric status, criminality and intelligence of 214 parents of these battered babies and 76 control parents. It also reports on the methods used by the Social Services Departments and the police in managing these 134 battered babies and their parents.

It is known that between 5 and 10 per cent of the general population exhibit EEG abnormalities (Hill and Watterson, 1942; Cobb, 1963). In more selected groups such as university students and flying personnel EEG abnormalities occur in less than 5 per cent (Williams, 1941; Harding, 1973). In contrast among those who are known to have commited acts of violence – for example, motiveless murder etc. – abnormalities may be found in 20 per cent or more (Hill, 1943; Stafford-Clark and Taylor, 1949). Because of this and because the author believed that insufficient emphasis has been placed upon the possible organic background of this type of anti-social behaviour it was also decided to undertake an investigation of EEG findings among baby batterers and any attendant abnormal personality correlates.

The importance of social adversities in precipitating baby battering have remained controversial. Some see the problem as a response to stressful social circumstances and society's permissive attitude to violence (Gil, 1970), others view it as primarily a manifestation of parental maladjustment (Steele and Pollock, 1968). A vast array of environmental stresses have also been regarded as contributory. Some have commented on the frequency of out-of-wedlock pregnancies (Simons *et al.*, 1966; Birrell and Birrell, 1968). A high incidence of divorce, separation and unstable marriages have also been reported (Kempe *et al.*, 1962). Social isolation, unemployment and lack of immediate support from other relatives are thought to be important (Young, 1964; Elmer, 1967). Other factors thought to be predisposing include, promiscuity (Young, 1964), larger than average family size (Gil, 1970), poverty, insufficient education (Galdston, 1965), geographical mobility (Gibbens and Walker, 1956; Schloesser, 1964) and inadequate housing (Birrell and Birrell, 1968). Paulson and Blake (1969) have cautioned against viewing battering parents as a function of educational, occupational and social disadvantage and have pointed out that most people in deprived sections of the community do not batter their children. In fact some regard social, educational, economic and demographic factors as irrelevant (Steele and Pollock, 1968); instead emphasis is laid on maladjustment resulting from harsh childhood experiences.

The foregoing chapters have outlined in detail the views of Morris and Gould (1963), Galdston (1965) and Steele and Pollock (1968). These and other authors have suggested that baby batterers were deprived of mothering in childhood and prematurely expect and demand a great deal from their own children. They also suggest that baby batterers have common misunderstandings with regard to child-rearing and look to the child for satisfaction of their own parental needs. Baby batterers are not, however, unique in this respect for the same is said to apply to murderers (MacDonald, 1963) and other criminals (Menninger, 1942).

Previous studies have not considered the issue that some factors may be typical of low social class populations and not particularly characteristic of baby batterers. Nor has the relative importance of various social stresses, childhood backgrounds and methods of child-rearing been adequately assessed. This study attempts to reconcile diverging opinions by examining a wide variety of such characteristics and the role of social class. It also aims to determine whether parents who confess to battering differ in certain respects from those who do not confess. A follow-up survey was also attempted and preliminary results are described in Chapter 16.

RESEARCH DESIGN

SUBJECTS

INDEX CASES

Over a period of 2 years 134 battered infants and children under 5 years of age and their parents were studied in detail. All their parents had either confessed to battering or could give no adequate explanation of their child's injuries and were referred to the author.

Ninety-one (68 per cent) were referred from eight hospitals in the West Midlands (*see* Table 4). Eighteen (13 per cent) were prison cases (their parents being convicted for battering their child who was hospitalized elsewhere. Twenty-five (19 per cent) came from other

TABLE 4
Hospitals Referring Battered Baby Cases (N = 91)

Birmingham Children's	59
Birmingham Accident	10
*{Wolverhampton Royal	7
{Dudley Guest	4
Selly Oak	4
Dudley Road	4
Warwick	2
East Birmingham	1

*The same consultant paediatrician was responsible for the paediatric wards of both hospitals.

sources: Social Services Departments, General Practitioners and Health Visitors.

CONTROL GROUP

The controls comprised 53 children under 5 years of age who were emergency admissions to Birmingham Children's Hospital and where there was no question of battering. Accident and trauma cases were excluded. Parents of these children were matched with the index group on the basis of the mother's age, and the age of the infant. The following variables were also held constant; consultants referring cases; area of residence (*see Figure 5)*; research team and the particular circumstances of the involvement of parents in research when their children suddenly and unexpectedly became ill. The problem of finding a control sample of equally low social class to match the index cases was impracticable (*see Figure 6*). However, it was possible to weight the index sample results equating them for social class of the controls (Newson, 1973*a*). This made it possible to determine whether abnormalities in the index sample were as significant when class was held constant. (Appendix C describes the statistical technique adopted.)

PROCEDURE

All parents were seen as soon as possible after the child's admission to hospital and their co-operation was requested in a research study into the background of children with injuries or conditions similar to that of their own child. (Appendix A describes the procedure in detail.) Both index and control parents underwent standardized psychiatric ,

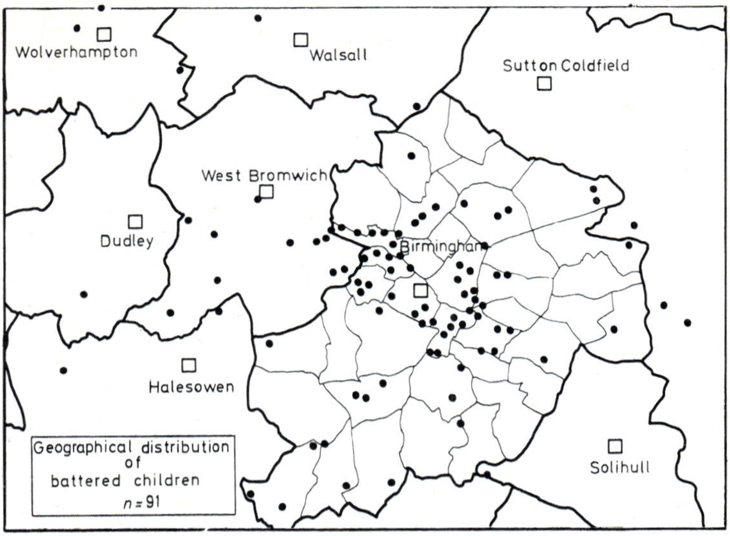

Figure 5. Map of Birmingham and surrounding districts showing approximate position of residence of battered children

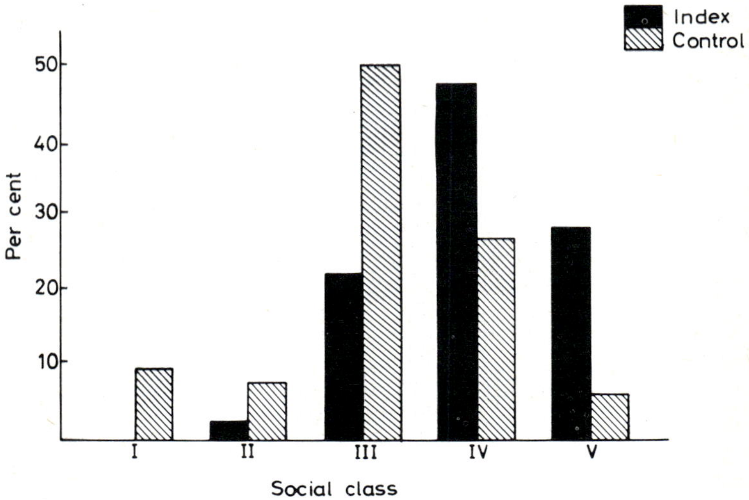

Figure 6. Comparison of social class distribution in index and control groups

psychological and social interviews. In the social interview, initial questions covered child-rearing practices, and subsequently family constitution, occupation, ethnic and religious background, financial circumstances and mother's attitude to the pregnancy and the child in this order. Accommodation, social life and marriage were covered next, and finally enquiry was made into satisfaction with life in general and into significant worries.(The interview schedules used are available to interested readers from the author.)

The general health and behaviour of the child and his siblings were recorded by a standardized medical interview. The medical notes were examined and the extent of the injuries recorded. All survivors were photographed and underwent full blood counts and skeletal surveys. Birth weights were recorded from maternity hospital notes. Family doctors were asked to examine their records; 84 were contacted, the remainder having no doctor. Forty-eight (57 per cent) replied.

The child's social maturation was measured by the Vineland Social Maturity Scale (Doll, 1947). The subscales (locomotor development, personal—social behaviour, hearing and speech, hand—eye co-ordination and performance) on the Griffiths Developmental Scale (Griffiths, 1954) were given to all children whose physical condition did not obviously entail brain damage. The child's social precocity was measured by calculating the discrepancy between the standard scores on the Vineland Social Maturity Scale and the Griffiths Developmental Scale (Pringle, 1969).

The EEGs of 35 subjects, who either confessed to inflicting injuries on their children or in whom the index of suspicion was high enough to make it virtually certain that they had done so were recorded. In addition to these, 16 of their husbands and wives were also subjected to EEG examination. In 13 other instances there was either no spouse or he or she was not available. Five failed to co-operate while one other who attended, fainted leading to abandonment of the procedure.

CLASSIFICATION

Personality diagnosis was classified on the basis of the American Psychiatric Association classification (1952) into normal and abnormal. Abnormality of personality was further subdivided into mild, moderate and severe.

Mild (character disorder)

Personality is disordered to the extent that the person is dissatisfied with the quality of his relationships with other people. Such persons may think they cannot make satisfying contacts with others owing to emotional inhibition, dependence on others or because of their own overbearing behaviour.

Moderate (personality disorder)

Impaired personal relationships are sufficiently noticeable to be evident to others. Such persons are perceived as unusual, odd or eccentric.

Severe (psychopathic)

Personality disorder is so gross that the subject harms others either through commission of aggressive acts or through omission of ordinary obligations. Thus psychopaths may be classified as aggressive or inadequate. Their work record is often poor (Walton and Presly, 1973).

The EEGs were divided into two groups. Those graded as normal either consisted of alpha activity with negligible amounts of theta activity (*see Figure* 7), or showed only low voltage beta activity. Those graded as *abnormal* contained noticeable theta activity, in the absence of drowsiness, though with some alpha activity (*see Figure 8*) or showed a dominant activity of low frequency or the presence of marked asymmetry (*see Figures 9* and *10*) or transient or complex activity of the type associated with epilepsy.

In all cases assessment of the EEG findings and psychiatric interviews were done 'blind', that is, each assessment was made without knowledge of the results of the other and the electro-encephalographer did not know whether the patient undergoing the EEG was the baby batterer or a spouse.

OTHER FACTORS

Neurosis was diagnosed at psychiatric interview and classified according to the International Classification of Disease (World Health Organization, 1968). Non-psychotic disturbance was measured by the General Health Questionnaire (Goldberg, 1972). Subjects scoring 12 or over on this scale have a high probability of being diagnosed as abnormal. Neuroticism (instability) was measured by the Eysenck Personality Inventory (Eysenck and Eysenck, 1964). Four subtests of the Wechsler Adult

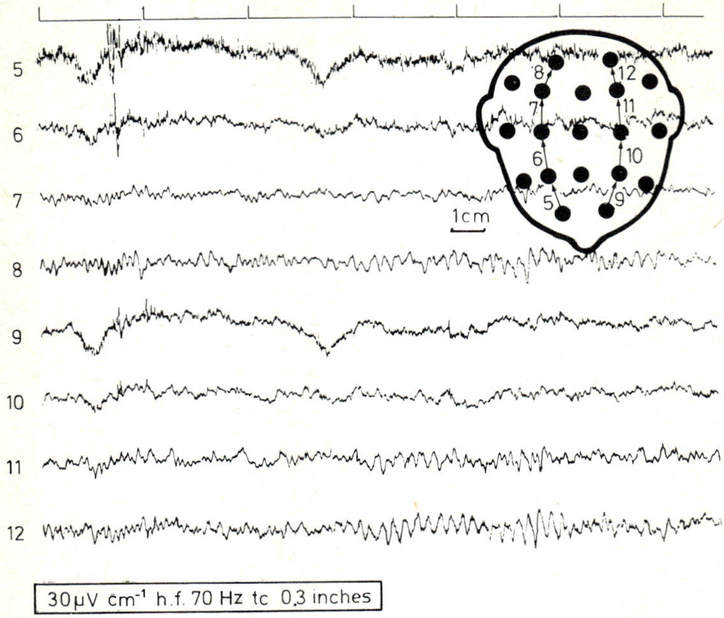

Figure 7. Normal EEG showing alpha activity and small amounts of theta activity

Intelligence Scale (Wechsler, 1955) were given (vocabulary, block design, comprehension and picture arrangement). Hostility was measured by Foulds Hostility and Direction of Hostility Questionnaire (Caine, Foulds and Hope, 1967). Psychomotor performance was measured by the Gibson Spiral Maze (Gibson, 1965). (A description of the tests used, the reasons for using them, and the order in which they were given is provided in Appendix A.)

A variety of difficulties the parents experienced with the child and spouse were explored by a specifically designed 'Difficult Times' test. The emotional reactions experienced by the parents when such difficulties arose were measured by a semantic differential technique. (Appendix B describes in detail these measures and the method of scoring the semantic differential. Some preliminary results obtained from a principal components analysis are also presented in this appendix.)

The Criminal Records Office was searched for the names of parents interviewed.

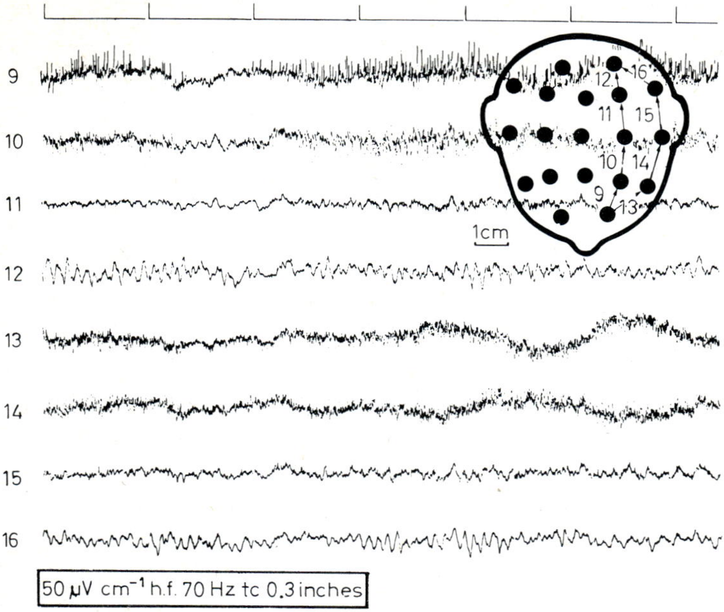

Figure 8. Abnormal EEG showing noticeable theta activity

DATA ANALYSIS

Analysis of data collected in this study focused on discerning associations between the phenomenon of baby battering and selected characteristics of battered children, their families, perpetrators of abuse and the circumstances surrounding abuse.

Following the interviews with both index and control groups, variables were coded and the data transferred to punch cards. The bulk of the required tabulations were carried out with the aid of the University of London Computer Centre using the Statistical Package for the Social Sciences (Nie, Bent and Hodlaihull, 1970).

Figure 11 demonstrates how the data was analysed. The following statistical techniques were applied to the data:

(1) Frequency counts and percentages on all variables for index and control groups. Mothers, fathers and children were analysed separately.

(2) For comparisons between groups and significance levels of

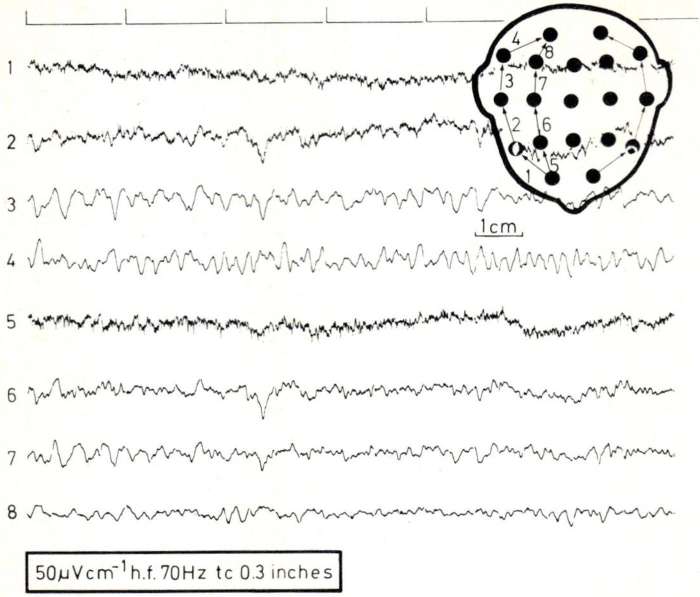

Figure 9. Abnormal EEG showing dominant activity of low frequency

differences, χ^2, with Yate's correction where applicable were used. (Appendix C gives questions and response categories which are not self evident in the approximate order in which results appear in the text). For numerical data, student's t test (based on separate variance estimates and two-tailed probabilities) were used.

(3) For associations, χ^2 contingency coefficients and Pearson's product moment correlations were used.

In assessing the significance of the results, only values of $p < 0.05$ (and $p < 0.01$) have been accepted as significant. Values of $p < 0.001$ have been accepted as highly significant.

Figure 11 also demonstrates how the results in this study are presented. The results compare index and control groups before and after adjustments were made for social class. The study also examined the results on all variables for known perpetrators and observed whether the perpetrators differed from the total sample. Tests of significance were carried out between the known perpetrators and those who were not

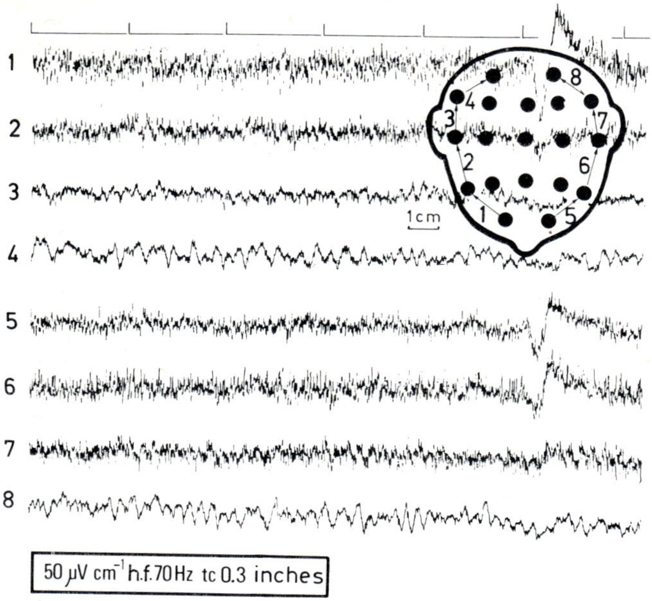

Figure 10. Abnormal EEG showing marked asymmetry

identified as such. Because many of the social characteristics – derived mainly from Part 2 of the Social Worker's schedule (*see* Appendix A) – applied to both parents, results for this section of the data have been given for mother and father perpetrators combined.

Chapter 11

Clinical Characteristics of the Children

SEX AND AGE OF CHILDREN

Sixty-eight (51 per cent) were boys and 66 (49 per cent) were girls. One hundred and ten (82 per cent) were under 2 years of age (mean age 18.5 months). *Figure 12* shows the age distribution of battered children. Emergency admissions were significantly younger than non-emergency admissions to Birmingham Children's Hospital ($\chi^2 = 79.30$; d.f. = 4; $p < 0.001$), (*see Figure 13*). Battered children were significantly younger than all other emergency admissions to the same hospital during 1971 ($\chi^2 = 9.5$; d.f. = 4; $p < 0.05$). *Figure 14* shows the sites of various injuries and the age of the children when these injuries were detected.

BRUISES, BURNS AND SCALDS

Thirty-eight (28 per cent) presented with conditions other than injuries. One hundred and ten (82 per cent) had bruises, most frequently on the head, 75 (56 per cent) and thighs, 45 (34 per cent). Twenty-three (17 per cent) had burns or scalds; in nine the buttocks and in six the lower limbs were affected. Injuries were most commonly caused by hot liquids or a metal stove. Cigarette burns occurred in two cases. Children with burns or scalds were significantly older (mean age 24.8 months) than the remainder of the sample ($t = 2.35$; $p < 0.05$), (*see Figure 15*).

FRACTURES

Forty-two (31 per cent) had recent or old fractures. The sites were

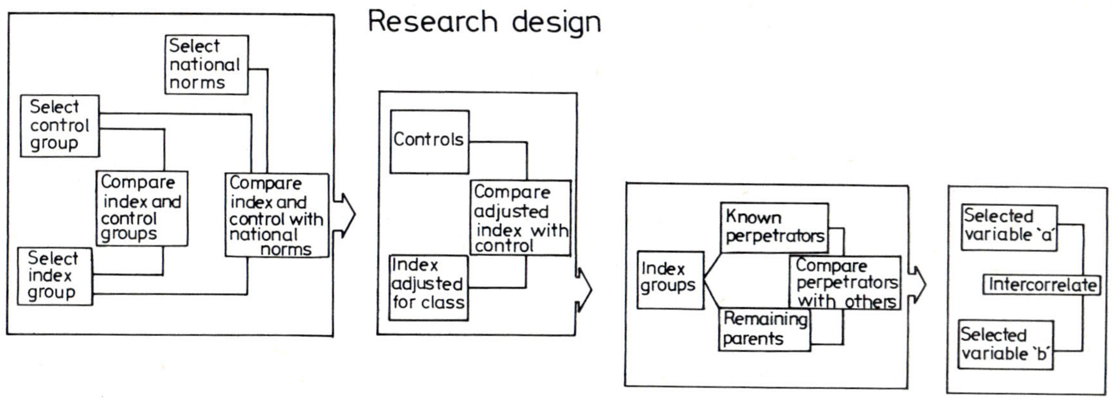

Figure 11. Schematic representation of research design and stages of analysis

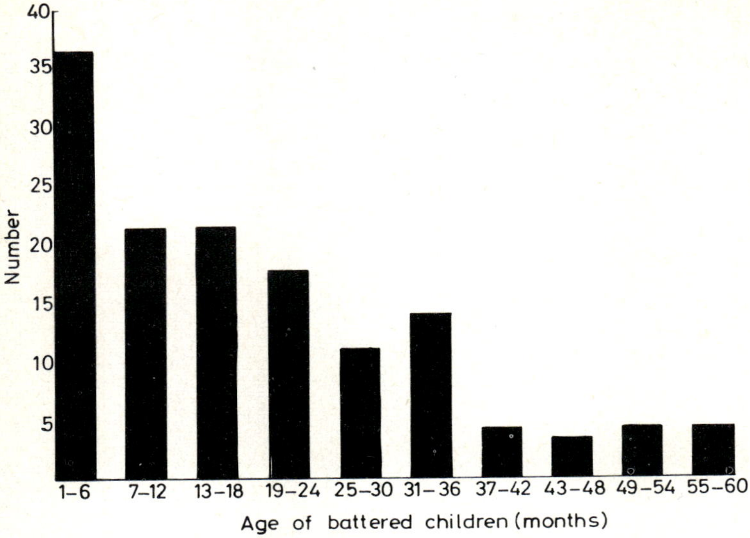

Figure 12. Age distribution of battered children

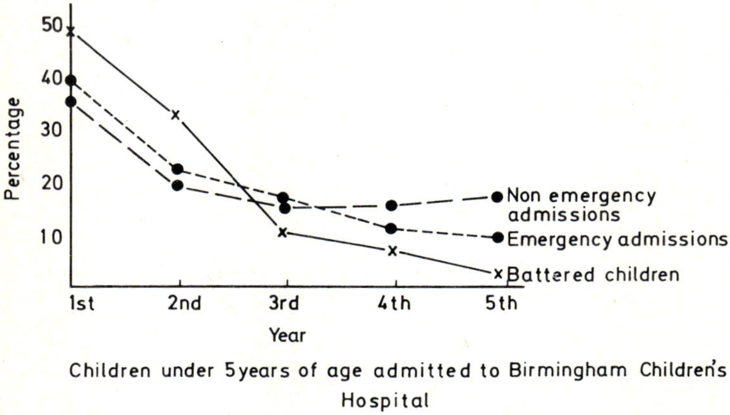

Figure 13. Age distribution of battered children compared with other emergency and non-emergency hospital admissions

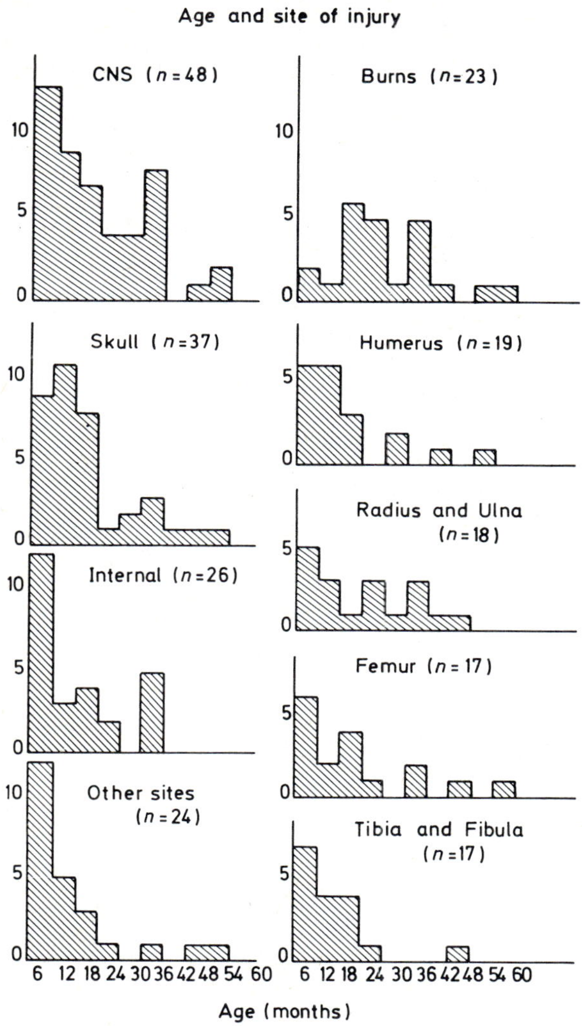

Figure 14. Sites of various injuries and the age of the children when these injuries were detected

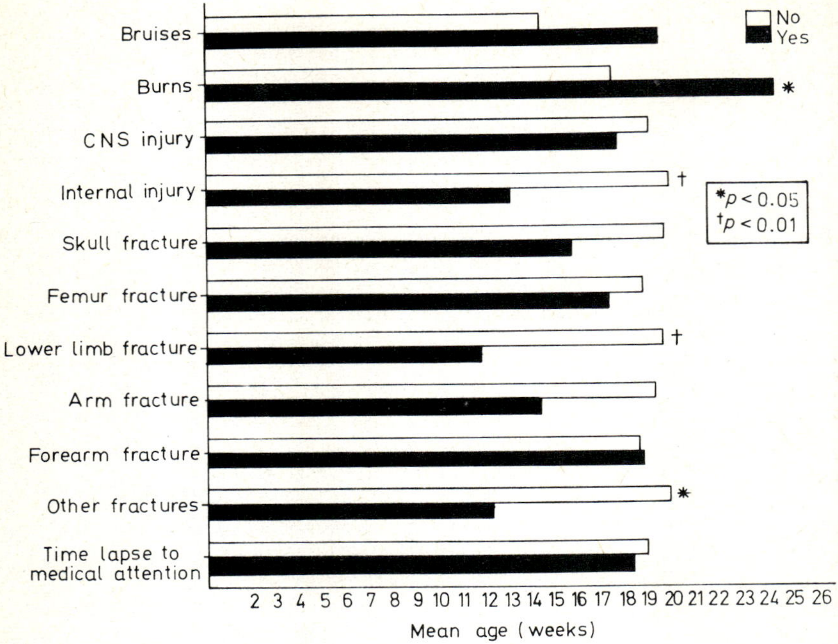

Figure 15. Injuries related to mean age

skull (37 cases), humerus (19 cases), radius and ulna (18 cases), femur (17 cases), tibia and fibula (17 cases), other sites (28 cases). Among those with burns 11 also had a fracture.

Children with lower limb and other fractures (ribs, scapulae) were significantly younger than the remainder of the sample (*see Figure 15*).

INTRACRANIAL AND INTRA-OCULAR HAEMORRHAGE

Forty-seven (35 per cent) had an intracranial haemorrhage. The types were subdural 30 cases (22 per cent), subarachnoid 9 cases (7 per cent), and cerebral 8 cases (6 per cent). Fifteen of these had no skull fractures and 7 no head bruises. Of the total sample 8 cases (6 per cent) had ocular damage in the form of intra-ocular haemorrhages, exudates, papilloedema or retinal detachments.

SERIOUSNESS OF INJURY

Twenty-one (16 per cent) children died. Twenty (15 per cent) had serious injuries resulting in permanent damage, 62 cases (46 per cent) serious injuries but no apparent damage and 31 cases (23 per cent) superficial injuries.

Fifty-nine cases (72 per cent) required hospitalization for up to 1 week, 16 cases (20 per cent) for 2–4 weeks and 7 cases (9 per cent) for 5 weeks or more. Forty-eight cases (36 per cent) remained in hospital for non-medical reasons for at least 1 additional week and 7 stayed for at least 5 weeks.

Dead children had significantly more skull fractures, central nervous system and internal injuries (ruptured viscera, peritonitis and intracranial haemorrhages) than the remainder (*see Figure 16*). A larger proportion also had another sibling who had been previously battered. There were 6 cases (33 per cent) of these compared with 25 cases (19 per cent) of live children. Seven cases (33 per cent) dead children compared with

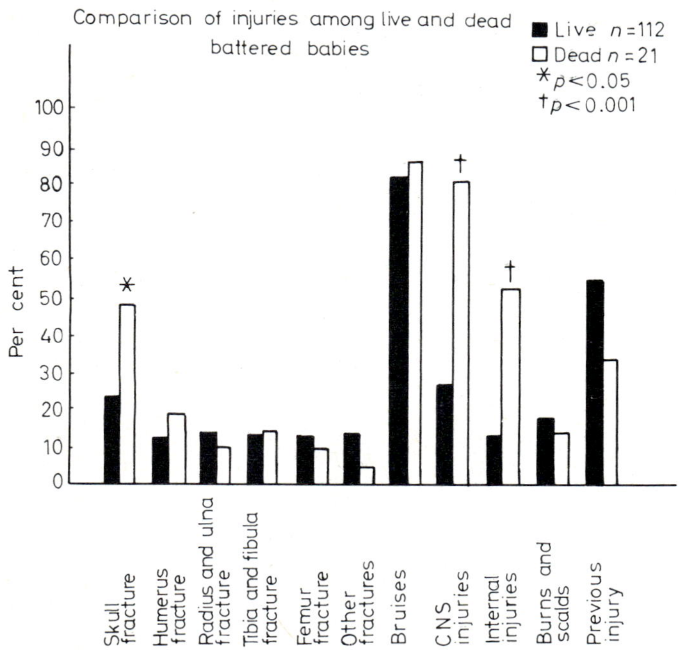

Figure 16. Comparison of injuries among those children who died from their injuries and those who did not

65 cases (50 per cent) of the rest had been battered more than once. Neither difference was significant. Among their parents 12 were convicted of either murder or manslaughter. In 9 cases the coroner reached an 'open verdict' and these parents were not prosecuted.

ABILITIES OF CHILDREN

Table 5 shows the suitability of children for mental developmental testing.

TABLE 5
Suitability of Children for Testing
(Griffiths Developmental Scales)

	No.	*Per cent of sample*
Untestable because of permanent damage	41	31
Recovered from head injury	36*	27
No head injury other than bruising	51	38
Not available for testing	6	4

* Includes four cases whose results were excluded because of serious congenital defects.

The mean general quotients on the Griffiths Scales were 89 for the index and 97 for control children ($t = 2.79$; $p < 0.01$). Excluding those who recovered from their head injuries the contrast between battered children and controls was of smaller significance ($t = 2.03$; $p < 0.05$). Mean general quotients for battered children with head injuries from which they had clinically recovered and those without head injuries were 87 and 90 respectively.

Figure 17 shows that battered children tested after head injury scored significantly lower than the controls on personal–social, hearing and speech, and hand–eye co-ordination scales. There were no significant differences between battered children who were not head injured and controls on the personal–social or hand–eye scales; only hearing and speech quotients were significantly lower for this subgroup of the battered sample.

Within the battered sample the mean developmental quotients of those with low birth weight was 73 and for those with failure to thrive 78.

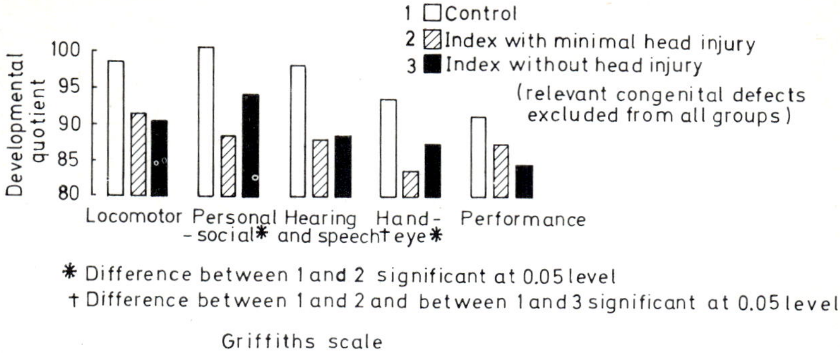

Figure 17. Griffiths Developmental Quotients among battered and control samples

SOCIAL MATURITY OF THE CHILD

The scores of 11 battered (15 per cent) compared with 3 controls (8 per cent) were one or more standard deviations higher on the Vineland Social Maturity Scale than on the Griffiths Developmental Quotient (difference not significant). Twelve battered (16 per cent) and 4 control children (11 per cent) were one or more standard deviation lower on the Vineland than on the Griffiths (this difference was also not significant). The Vineland scores correlated with the Griffiths quotients in the index sample (C = 0.58) and among the controls (C = 0.80).

PHYSICAL NEGLECT AND FAILURE TO THRIVE

Twenty-two battered children (17 per cent) compared with 1 control (2 per cent) were physically neglected on admission ($\chi^2 = 6.51$; d.f. = 1; $p < 0.05$) and 23 battered children (17 per cent) compared with 1 control (2 per cent) had previously been in hospital with failure to thrive ($\chi^2 = 6.62$; d.f. = 1; $p < 0.01$). Among the battered children failure to thrive occurred in 11 (50 per cent) of the neglected children and 11 (10 per cent) of the remainder ($\chi^2 = 17.64$; d.f. = 1; $p < 0.001$).

BIRTH WEIGHT

Of the battered children born in hospital 58 (75 per cent) had normal birth weights, 8 (10 per cent) weighed between 2000 and 2500 g, and

11 (14 per cent) weighed less than 2000 g. The occurrence of low birth weight among the different social classes is shown in Table 6 and compared with national norms (Drillien, 1964; Wadsworth, 1974). In both upper and lower social classes the prevalence of low birth weight among the battered sample born in hospital was four times greater than the national rate.

TABLE 6
Percentage of Low Birth Weight Babies
(less than 2500 g) according to Social Class in Three Studies

<table>
<tr><th>Social class</th><th>Drillien</th><th>Smith and Hanson</th><th>National Survey of Health and Development (Wadsworth)</th></tr>
<tr><td>I and II</td><td>3.3</td><td rowspan="2">24</td><td rowspan="2">5.6</td></tr>
<tr><td>III</td><td>5.9</td></tr>
<tr><td>IV and V</td><td>7.6</td><td>24</td><td></td></tr>
</table>

NUMBER OF DECEASED SIBLINGS

Ten battered children (9 per cent) had a deceased sibling. Four of these had died under 'suspicious' circumstances. In two cases more than one sibling had died. None of the controls had a deceased sibling.

CONGENITAL DEFECTS

Altogether 10 of the battered children (7.46 per cent) had serious congenital defects as compared with 1.75 per cent of the general population (Butler and Alberman, 1969). There were 2 cases each of spina bifida, hydrocephalus, and encephalocele and 1 each of Hirschsprung's disease, coeliac disease, congenital spherocytosis, and congenital dislocation of the hip. A further 8 children had minor congenital abnormalities.

PRECIPITANTS

Eighty mothers (60 per cent) and 63 fathers (71 per cent) initially denied inflicting injury but gave no adequate explanation of it. Thirteen mothers (10 per cent) and 6 fathers (6 per cent) later changed their initial account into an adequate explanation of the injury. Among mothers, 16 (12 per cent) had had a confinement less than 3 months previously, 56 (42 per cent) between 3 and 12 months previously and 62 (46 per cent) more than 12 months before the battering incident.

Crying was reported as a precipitant by 20 mothers (21 per cent) and 13 fathers (34 per cent). Among mothers 26 (25 per cent) reported that the child was doing something naughty for which he had been previously forewarned. Battering incidents occurred equally in the morning 35 (33 per cent) and late afternoon 36 (34 per cent). Thirty-one (29 per cent) occurred in the evening. Only 5 parents (5 per cent) reported they battered the child late at night.

BEHAVIOUR OF CHILD AND NEUROTICISM OF MOTHERS

Table 7 shows that battered children were significantly less wakeful at night, excitable or lively, or tired during the day, than the controls. No significant differences were found on time of rising or going to bed or poor appetite. One child who failed to thrive was considered by its mother to have a feeding problem, compared with 14 of those who did thrive. The difference was not significant.

TABLE 7
Comparison between Behaviour at Home of Battered Children and Control Children

	Battered Children		*Control*		*Significance*	
	No.	*Per cent*	*No.*	*Per cent*	χ^2	p
Wakeful at night (0.5 hr or longer)	11/123	(9)	11/51	(22)	4.12	< 0.05
Excitable or lively	76/125	(61)	40/51	(78)	4.26	< 0.05
Tired during day	49/124	(39)	31/51	(61)	5.76	< 0.05
Rose 5–7 a.m.	38/123	(31)	16/51	(31)	0.01	N.S.
Went to bed 9–12 p.m.	30/123	(24)	15/51	(29)	0.25	N.S.
Poor appetite	15/124	(12)	7/51	(14)	0.00	N.S.
Crying a problem	39/107	(36)	4/48	(8)	11.49	< 0.001

Forty (30 per cent) mothers of battered children compared with 5 (9 per cent) control mothers considered the child difficult ($\chi^2 = 8.40$; d.f. = 1; $p < 0.01$). Of the 40 mothers 30 (75 per cent) were neurotic whereas only 29 (31 per cent) of those who did not find their children difficult were ($\chi^2 = 16.21$; d.f. = 1; $p < 0.001$). Thirty-six (27 per cent) mothers of battered children compared with 4 (8 per cent) control mothers described their other children as difficult ($\chi^2 = 14.12$; d.f. = 1; $p < 0.001$). More (39; 29 per cent) mothers of battered children – of whom 27 (69 per cent) were neurotic – than control mothers (4; 8 per cent) said crying, clinging, or whining behaviour was a severe problem ($\chi^2 = 11.49$; d.f. = 1; $p < 0.001$). Fewer of the mothers who did not find such behaviour a problem were neurotic – only 29 (31 per cent) ($\chi^2 = 7.51$; d.f. = 1; $p < 0.01$). The proportion of mothers reporting messy, destructive behaviour, temper tantrums and disobedience was not significantly higher than among the controls.

DELAY IN ATTENDING HOSPITAL AND PREVIOUS CONTACT WITH GENERAL PRACTITIONERS

The parents of 82 battered children (61 per cent) attended the hospital casualty department at least 24 hours after injury occurred. Eleven children (53 per cent) with serious injuries (including some who later died from their injuries) were also presented after similar delay. According to the family doctor's reports, no parent had made unnecessary visits. According to their own reports 113 (87 per cent) had rarely or never consulted their general practitioner prior to battering their child.

Chapter 12

Case Reports and Clinical Illustrations

CASE 1

The following case description illustrates the importance of early diagnosis of unexplained injuries and the difficulties confronting those who have to ensure the child's safety. Efforts to rehabilitate battering parents should not be at the expense of the safety of the child. This case suggests that a care order on other children in a family, even though not yet battered, should be strongly considered.

A boy aged 2 years, asleep in a pram outside a store was seen by a passing policewoman to have a black eye. On inquiry, the mother of the child informed the policewoman that the child received the injury after a fall. The mother had not taken the child to a doctor because she did not think it necessary as the child was always having 'accidents'. However, she agreed with the policewoman that the child should be immediately examined and accompanied her to the nearby hospital casualty department. Examination at the hospital revealed the child to have additional injuries (*see Plates 1, 2* and *3* in plate section facing page 140). Evidence of minimal but older bruising over the back was said to have occurred when the boy 'walked backwards into a door handle'; an old burn across the flexure of the knee was due to the child 'walking backwards into an electric fire'. A skeletal survey revealed an old fractured wrist, consistent in the radiologist's opinion, with rough handling – this was denied by the mother. Because of the inadequately explained nature of these injuries the child was admitted to hospital. Other medical conditions which may possibly have accounted for his injuries were excluded. During his stay on the ward it was observed he sustained no further injuries.

A case conference was held and the social services department assured the paediatricians that the child's safety could be supervised on a voluntary basis, and that the parents would bring the child at regular intervals to the hospital for re-assessment. Over the next few weeks, however, the parents failed to keep several appointments. The social worker managing the case reassured the doctors that he had visited the home and seen that the child was progressing well.

Seven weeks after the boy's discharge from hospital, his sister, aged 9 months, was admitted to the same hospital with a haematoma over the scalp and an extensively fractured skull. Both parents 'thought' that the child had fallen from a pram. A second case conference was called, at which the hospital staff were again reassured that the child's safety could be guaranteed by supervision and that it was not necessary to remove these children into care. As a 'precautionary' measure, however, it was decided to bring the case to the attention of the juvenile court. The magistrates were presented with medical evidence that left no doubt that the girl's injuries were very inadequately explained. Information relating to her brother's earlier admission to hospital and the psychiatric opinion that it would be hazardous to return these children home, was not presented. It was not surprising, therefore, that the doctors were disconcerted when they learned that the magistrates had followed the recommendation of the social services department and issued a supervision order on the girl.

Two weeks after the juvenile court hearing, the little girl was examined in the casualty department with multiple intra-abdominal injuries and peritonitis. She died in hospital shortly after admission as a result of these extensive injuries. Despite a pathologist stating at the inquest that these injuries were undoubtedly caused by a series of blows, an 'open' verdict was reached by the coroner. The parents denied inflicting injury and the police did not proceed with prosecution because of 'lack of evidence'. Following the death of the child, her brother was taken into care.

CASE 2

The following case describes an anorexia nervosa mother who battered her elder male child and in collusion with her psychopathic husband starved to death her daughter aged 10 weeks. This case illustrates the dangers of focusing on a battered child without regard to its siblings; the battered child was closely supervised by a health visitor and social worker who both failed to notice the development of marasmus in his younger sister. Though this case is unusual it does, however, illustrate the association between baby battering and failure to thrive and underlines the importance of a psychiatric assessment of the parents.

Mrs. P when first seen was aged 22 years. In August 1967 she was involved in an automobile accident. Her injuries were not severe consisting of minor bruising, abrasions and lacerations over her body but not her head. Following this she developed loss of confidence and a phobia of driving or being driven. In June 1968 she was referred to a consultant neurologist complaining of frequent 'blackouts', general nervousness and loss of weight from 69.3 to 48.0 kg and marked loss of appetite. Although she did not actually suffer from amenorrhoea her periods were very scanty, consisting of a relatively slight loss lasting a day or two and occurring every 19 days. Physical examination revealed a very thin woman but with no other abnormal physical signs. Haematological and biochemical investigations were normal. Her EEG showed only a slight non-specific abnormality. A diagnosis of anorexia nervosa was made and the patient was referred to a consultant psychiatrist who concurred with this.

Her early development was normal apart from slight feeding difficulty in infancy. She reached a weight of 69.3 kg and 69 cm height during adolescence. Her school years were uneventful apart from occasional 'giddy turns'. On leaving she became a shop assistant.

In January 1968 she married. Her parents strongly objected to her choice of husband. He was 32 years of age, suffered from a squint and a stammer and had often been ridiculed at school. He later had several unskilled jobs, and was dismissed or made redundant from most of them. When seen he had not worked for 18 months, in order, he said, to look after his wife. He showed some features of an aggressive but inadequate psychopathic personality. There was no history of any psychiatric disorder in either the patient's or her husband's family.

In September 1969 Mrs. P. gave birth to a normal male infant weighing 3.1 kg. Labour and delivery were normal. Two months later it was noticed that the baby was undernourished with very little subcutaneous fat. Head bruising was noted several times by the health visitor and each time was inadequately explained. Both parents denied the baby was difficult to feed and denied inflicting trauma. However, they were extremely reluctant to allow the general practitioner and health visitor to examine the child. The child is still rather thin and appears retarded in development and some slight facial bruising is still seen on occasions.

In December 1970 Mrs. P gave birth to her second child, a female weighing 3.2 kg. Labour and delivery were normal and the baby fed well in hospital and shortly after discharge. Ten weeks later, however, the baby was admitted as an emergency following a visit by the health visitor who noticed she was extremely cold and underweight. Examination revealed an extremely emaciated, dehydrated and corpse-like child (*see Plates 4* and *5* in plate section facing page 140). Temperature was 25°C, weight 2.7 kg. She was anaemic and there was no pulse. She had an ulcerated nappy rash (*see Plate 6* in plate section facing page 140). A diagnosis of hypothermia and marasmus was made. Despite intensive efforts at resuscitation she died the following day. Necropsy revealed no evidence of bruising, fractures or internal injury. The failure to thrive was attributed to poor feeding. Neither parent could account for the rapid weight loss. They stated the baby was feeding well and denied starving or neglecting her in any way. A verdict of 'lack of care' was recorded.

Since the death of the baby Mrs. P has lost another stone in weight (present weight 42.7 kg). Mr. P is still not working and the family is living on social security benefits.

Intelligence, personality and attitude tests were given to Mrs. P 3 months after the death of her child. These showed an IQ of 84 (WAIS) and on the Eysenck Personality Inventory (EPI) an extremely high N score and an E score well above average. Her lie (L) score was very low. Her scores on the Hostility and Direction of Hostility Questionnaire showed her to be extremely hostile, chiefly towards other people but with considerable self-criticism and guilt.

An inquiry into difficulties around the time when her baby was alive showed that she had found the child extremely demanding. Scores on the Semantic Differential scale suggested moderate reactions to the child's attention-seeking, but very disturbed reactions, especially on the Sensitivity and Depression scales to problems with neighbours, which appear to have been present before the death of the child.

Her husband contradicted himself on questions relating to difficulties with the baby, and denied they were anything to do with his wife or outsiders. His responses to the Semantic Differential test were evasive. This is consonant with his high score on the L scale of the EPI where he gave a picture of an extremely stable, moderately extroverted person. On the Hostility Questionnaire he expressed an average amount of hostility, most of which was projected; there were no guilt feelings and practically no self-criticism. His I.Q. was 82.

COMMENTARY

One view of the cause of anorexia nervosa is that it represents a rejection by the patient of her mother (Hobhouse, 1938; Ross, 1938). Bruch (1966) drew attention to these patients' 'pursuit of thinness' while Crisp (1967) claimed that primary anorexia nervosa is a disorder which has as its basis a phobia of normal adolescent weight. Crisp has also described how certain of his anorexia nervosa patients who have recovered and gone on to have children have mentioned inability to feel affection for the child (Crisp, 1971).

Steele and Pollock (1968) have commented in their psychiatric study of parents of battered children that such parents have expectations of the child far beyond its chronological age. If no gratification of these expectations is received the parent responds with frustration and anger. In addition, the mother who does not receive adequate emotional support from her husband or parents and who has a difficult time with her pregnancy may feel the demands of child-rearing as overwhelming. If the child comes to represent someone to whom she herself expects to turn, she may look to the child for much of the understanding or support that is lacking in her present situation.

This case exemplifies the pattern. The patient was dependent on her husband who was unable to support her emotional needs, while her own parents disapproved of her marriage. It is possible that starving the younger girl may have been a substitute for battering her son, the passive behaviour in the first instance being a substitute for the more active in the past.

In any event the literature contains several references correlating failure to thrive and battering (Koel, 1969; Bullard *et al.*, 1967; Barbero and Shaheen, 1967). These studies have hypothesized that failure to thrive and battering of children are on a continuum. This case also illustrates this hypothesis.

CASE 3

The following case describes the onset of infantile spasms (West's syndrome) following trauma. Though the aetiology cannot be stated with certainty there is a strong probability that the child's symptoms were directly related to the mother shaking the infant. This case demonstrates that repeated acceleration/deceleration(whiplash injury) rather than direct violence may account for intracranial bleeding. It also illustrates the importance of considering maltreatment as a possible aetiological factor in those children with neurological disorders for which no adequate cause has been identified.

Lauren (d.o.b. 21.5.72) was the second child of a 24 year old mother. The mother's pregnancy was complicated by anaemia for which she received liver injections. The pregnancy was full-term and labour and delivery were normal. Lauren weighed 2.9 kg, breathed and cried well at birth and was well until the time of admission when aged 3 months.

Three days prior to admission the mother reported that Lauren went limp and her eyes rolled. Her mouth lay open and she made 'funny noises'. During this episode she vomited slightly and cried as she recovered. She was a little dazed in the evening, but seemed to be well the following day. Two days later she vomited and on the next day following a severe episode of vomiting she suddenly 'became lifeless'. There was some blood in the vomit. On this particular day the mother had observed that Lauren twitched on the right and then on the left. The family doctor was called and he prescribed penicillin. Following the first dose she again vomited and recommenced twitching and shortly after was admitted to hospital.

The mother felt that Lauren's development prior to these episodes had been normal. She thought Lauren was a quick developer, who looked around, gurgled, was able to hear, smiled and was a generally active child. She mentioned that Lauren occasionally had 'crying fits' when she sometimes went stiff and banged her face on the side of the cot. In general, however, she slept well. As far as the mother was aware, Lauren had never fallen, hurt herself or banged her head. There was no history of ingestion of non-food substances or any bleeding disorder.

On examination, the child was ill. Her head circumference was 41 cm (50th centile) and the fontanelle was flat and pulsating normally. She had a left-sided facial weakness. Her fundi showed massive subhyaloid haemorrhages with pale centres. There was a generalized increase in tone, more marked on the left than on the right side. There was no evidence of external bruising and other body systems appeared normal. A diagnosis of cerebral haemorrhage of unknown aetiology was made. Coagulation screening and a thorough search for infection yielded negative results. Cerebrospinal fluid was bloodstained with supernatant xanthochromia. The C.S.F. sugar was 80 mg per cent and revealed no organisms. An x-ray of the skull and skeletal survey showed no evidence of trauma.

Management comprised close observation and prophylactic phenobarbitone, with valium for the seizures if they were prolonged Over the next 48 hours the fontanelle increased in size and epidural taps confirmed the presence of fresh subdural haemorrhage. The combination of subdural and subarachnoid haemorrhages, together with subhyaloid and retinal haemorrhages in a previously normal child, strongly suggested a traumatic origin.

The nature of Lauren's injuries were outlined to the parents. The mother reported that prior to Lauren's admission to hospital she had become increasingly frustrated and irritable and had begun to handle her baby in a 'rough manner'. On several occasions she had shaken Lauren violently and had come very close to striking her. There was considerable tension within the household, particularly between Lauren's parents. This was largely due to Lauren's mother being unable to care for her son aged 3 years. This child had resulted from a casual acquaintance with a man who was not Lauren's father. Her husband's parents, with whom the family were living, refused to allow her 'illegitimate son' into their home. They also prevented her from visiting the boy who was being cared for by foster parents. Lauren's mother had also been ostracized by her own parents and had recently sought treatment for a depressive illness. She was finding the demands of rearing Lauren overwhelming. It was the consensus of professional opinion, that because the major cause of Lauren's trauma lay in the immediate home environment no legal proceedings should be instituted. Furthermore remedial action to correct the current adversities would do much to relieve the pressures on this mother.

PROGRESS

Initially Lauren did well and was discharged home aged 5 months. Her seizures completely disappeared, she was progressing in development and the only abnormal findings were brisk reflexes in the lower limbs and a suggestion of diminished cortical visual function. She was maintained on phenobarbitone 50 mg three times a day.

When 7 months old Lauren was presented to out-patients with a history of having been generally unwell for a few days – she was more drowsy than before. Her mother described episodes of spasms, during which Lauren flexed forward and the muscles of the abdomen became tense. The mother attributed these episodes to colic because Lauren cried out during these attacks. They occurred in groups of 4 or 5 at a time and in the few days prior to admission she had about half-a-dozen episodes. These attacks were somewhat different from the original attacks, which precipitated Lauren's first hospital admission. On examination the child showed no evidence of external bruising. The head circumference was 43 cms. The fontanelle was normal and there was no evidence of retinal haemorrhages. Lauren was, however, a little more hypotonic than she had been, but apart from this showed no new neurological signs. An EEG confirmed classical hypsarrhythmia with high amplitude mixture of slow waves at 1–3 cycles/sec, mixed with spikes. The abnormality was seen in all areas (*see Figure 18*).

Previous EEGs during the first admission showed no evidence of

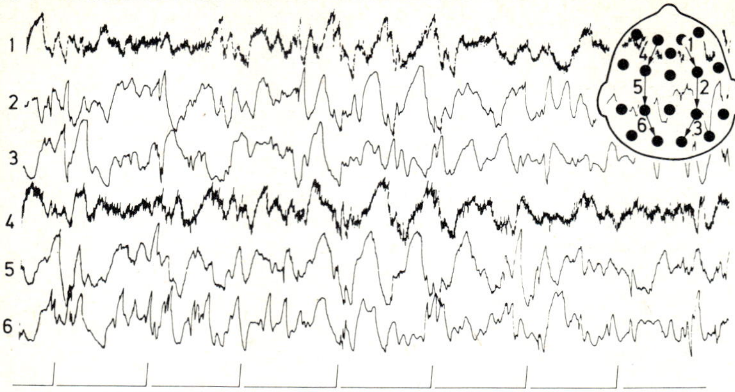

Figure 18. EEG of Lauren, Case 3, demonstrating hypsarrhythmia. (Medication, Phenobarbitone 15 mg b.d.)

This record shows a high amplitude mixture of slow waves at 1 – 3 c.p.s. mixed with spikes, the abnormality being seen in all areas. From time to time there is an increase in the spiking which is bilateral. This chaotic mixture was found to be continuous throughout the tracing. This record shows hypsarrhythmia and confirms the diagnosis of infantile spasms

hypsarrhythmia (*see Figure 19*). Lauren was, therefore, treated with ACTH, 40 units intramuscularly each day, for 7 days. Following this treatment the EEG was repeated and showed significant improvement (*see Figure 20*). Clinical improvement occurred concurrently and no

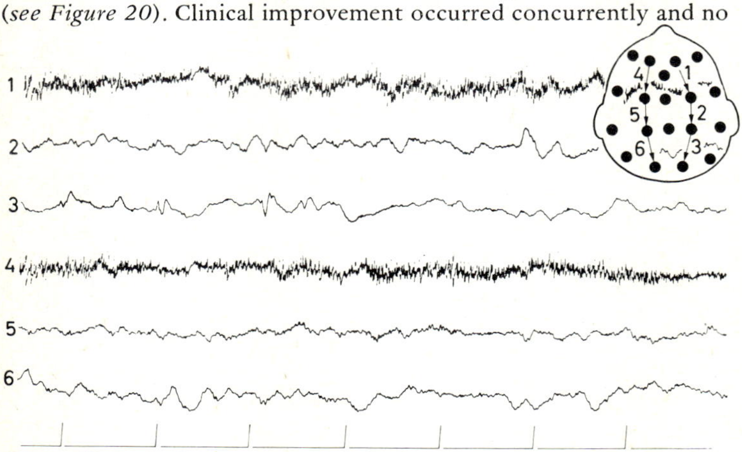

Figure 19. EEG of Lauren, Case 3, before the development of hypsarrhythmia. (Medication, Phenobarbitone 15 mg t.i.d.)

This record shows some abnormal slow wave activity which is more marked on the right than on the left and maximal in the occipital derivations. In addition there are occasional sharp waves on the right and also in the occipital derivation. This recording is consistent with the diagnosis and clinical history

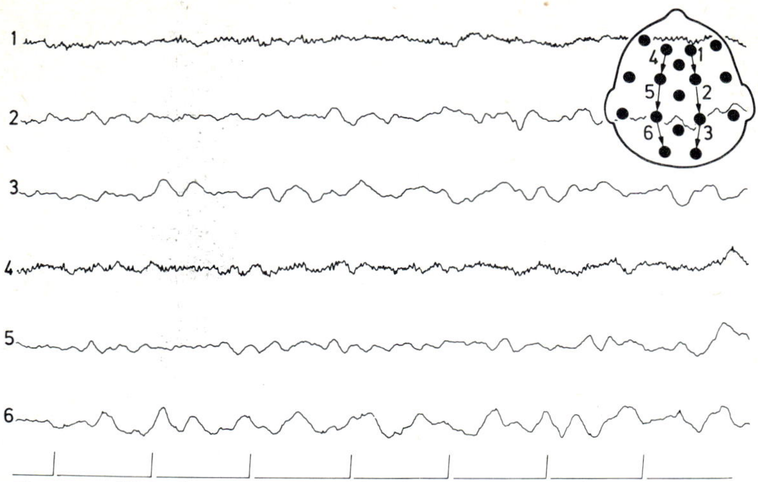

Figure 20. EEG of Lauren, Case 3, following treatment. (Medication ACTH 40 units per day).

This recording is dominated by bilateral slow activity at 2–4 c.p.s., the amplitude being slightly higher on the left than on the right. There are a few occasional discharges and photic stimulation evoked no abnormality. Though the record is a little slow there is no definite abnormality

further spasms occurred. Over a month, the ACTH was gradually tailed off and when Lauren was eight months old the EEG, apart from being little slow, was essentially normal. Since that time Lauren has been maintained on prednisone and nitrazepam. She has had no further spasms and her general development has improved.

COMMENT

West (1841) originally described a 'peculiar form of infantile convulsion' consisting of salaam spasms associated with mental retardation. More than a century elapsed, however, before the full syndrome – spasms, mental retardation and an abnormal EEG (hypsarrhythmia) – was documented (Vazquez and Turner, 1951, Gibbs and Gibbs, 1952).

The aetiology of the triad often remains undetermined but medical reports disclose, as one factor, an association with trauma particularly cerebral birth injury (Millichap *et al.*, 1962; Jeavons and Bower, 1974). Violent shaking as a form of child abuse may give rise to cerebral injury (Guthkelch, 1971; Caffey, 1972; Smith and Hanson, 1974) but there have been no recorded examples of infantile spasms following such an episode.

Though an infectious encephalopathy cannot be definitely excluded there is a strong probability that Lauren's spasms followed the cerebral injury. Furthermore, the nature of this injury, with evidence of intracranial bleeding suggested that this may have been produced by the whiplash effect of shaking (Guthkelch, 1971; Caffey, 1972). The syndrome of infantile spasms is associated with many pathological processes of which the commonest – accounting for at least one third of all cases – is perinatal brain damage (Jeavons and Bower, 1974). Considering that most baby batterers offer no adequate explanation for their child's injury (Smith and Hanson, 1974) and that approximately half the cases of cerebral palsy and mental deficiency attending paediatric out-patient departments have no adequate cause identified (MacKeith, 1974), the possibility that child abuse is responsible for a proportion of 'cryptogenic' cases of West's syndrome needs further exploration.

CLINICAL ILLUSTRATIONS

A summary of the principal sites and types of injuries observed in this study. *Figures 21–27* and *Plates 7–17* (*see* plate section facing page 140) illustrate some of these injuries and demonstrate the inadequately explained nature of some of them.

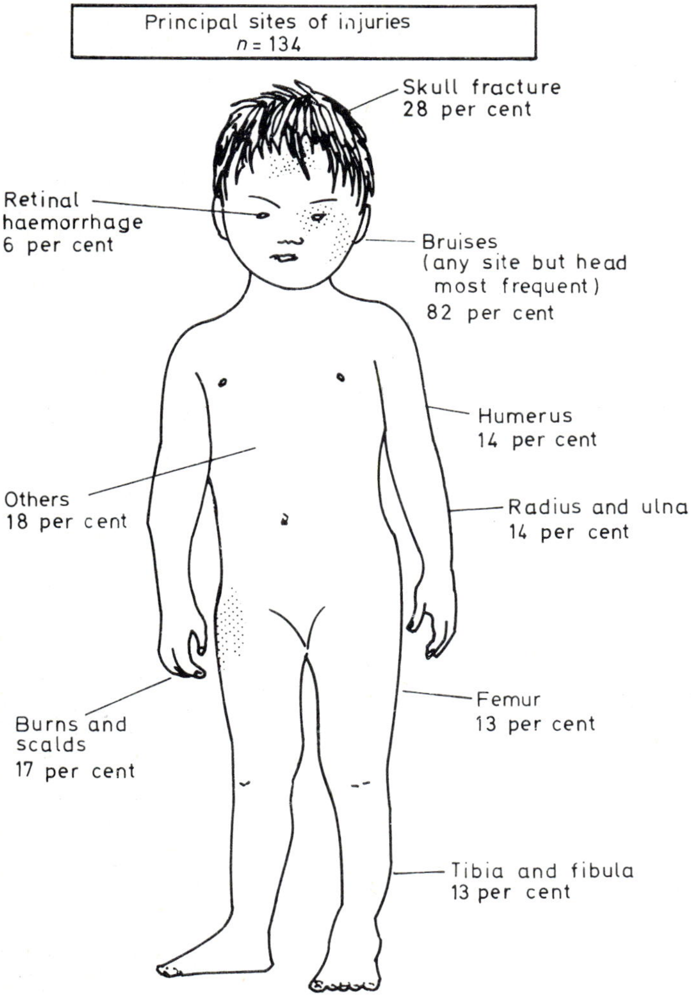

Figure 21. Demonstration of principal sites of injuries

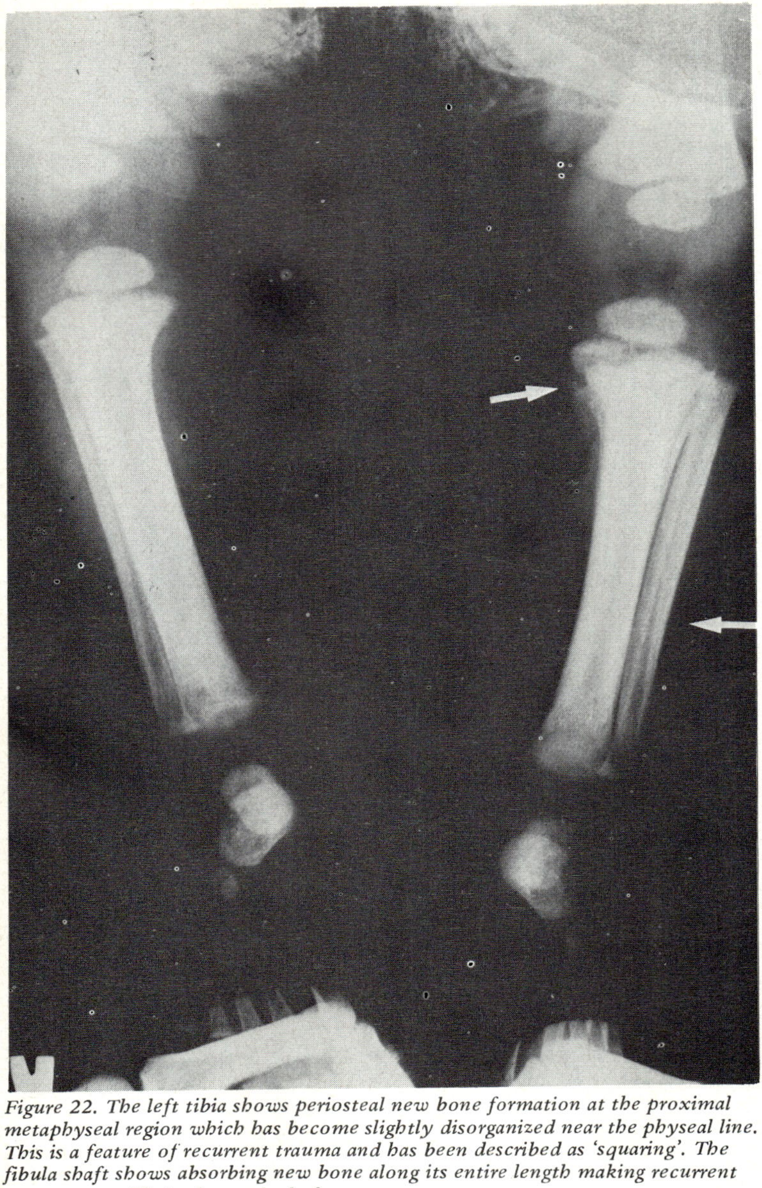

Figure 22. The left tibia shows periosteal new bone formation at the proximal metaphyseal region which has become slightly disorganized near the physeal line. This is a feature of recurrent trauma and has been described as 'squaring'. The fibula shaft shows absorbing new bone along its entire length making recurrent trauma more likely than a single fracture

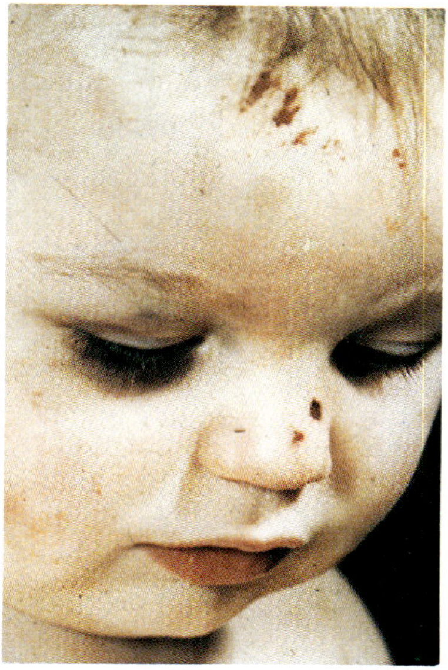

Plate 1. Boy aged 2 years, described in Case 1, showing abrasions, a 'black eye' and bruising of the right cheek, attributed by the parents to recurrent accidents

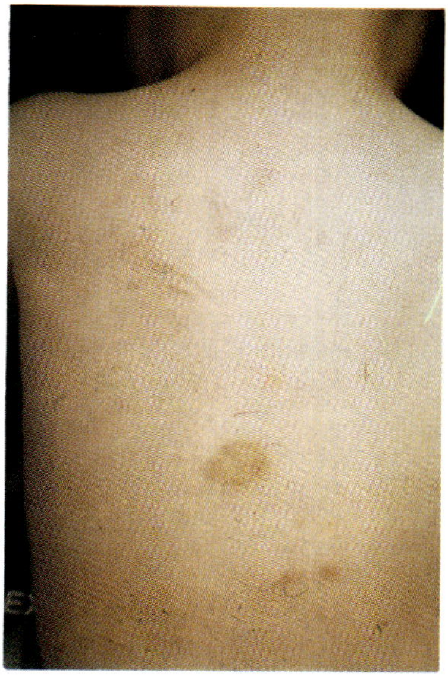

Plate 2. Same child as in Plate 1, showing minimal bruising to the back attributed by the parents to 'walking backwards into a door handle'

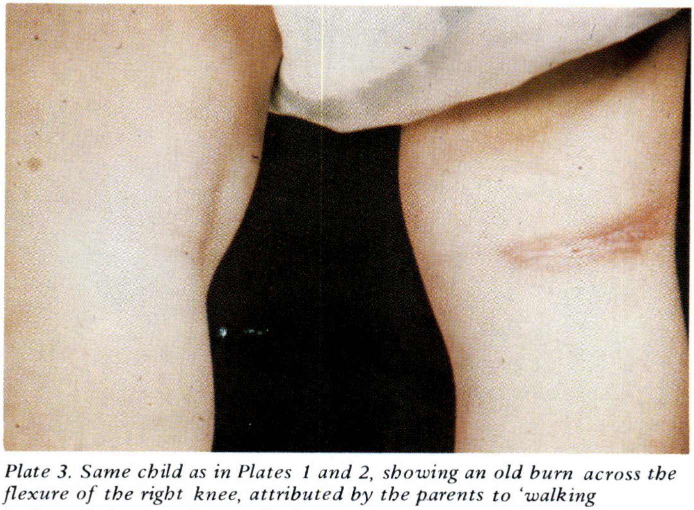

Plate 3. Same child as in Plates 1 and 2, showing an old burn across the flexure of the right knee, attributed by the parents to 'walking backwards into an electric fire'

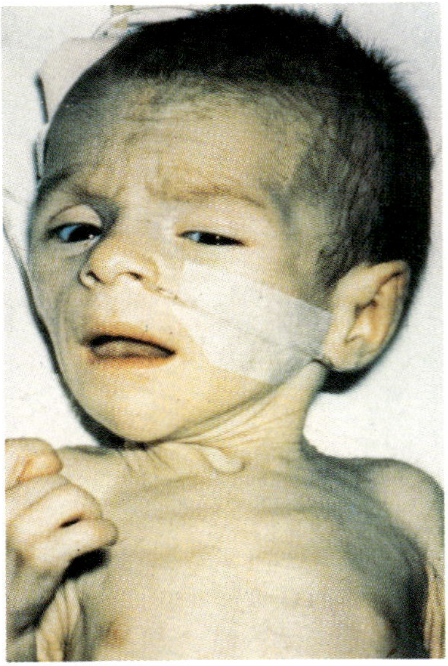

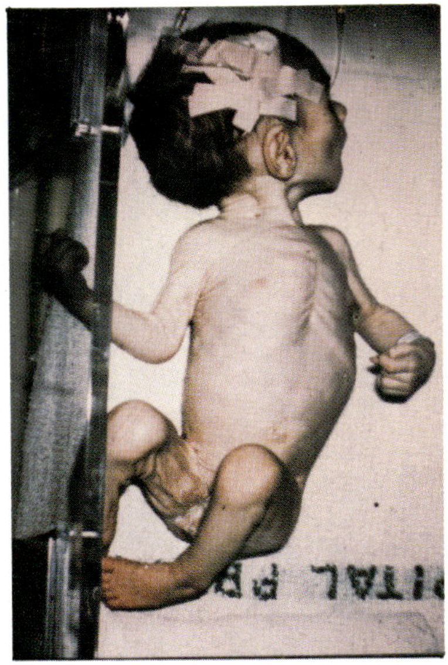

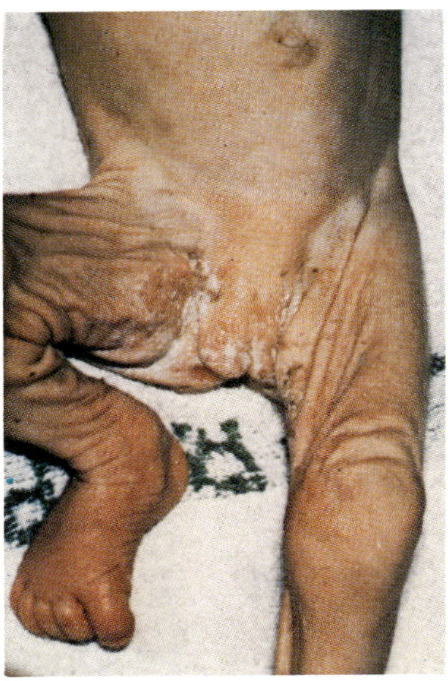

Plate 4. Female aged 10 weeks, described in Case 2, showing extreme emaciation and dehydration

Plate 5. Same child as in Plate 4. These photographs were taken 2 hours after admission to hospital

Plate 6. Same child as in Plates 4 and 5 showing ulcerated nappy rash and marked dehydration

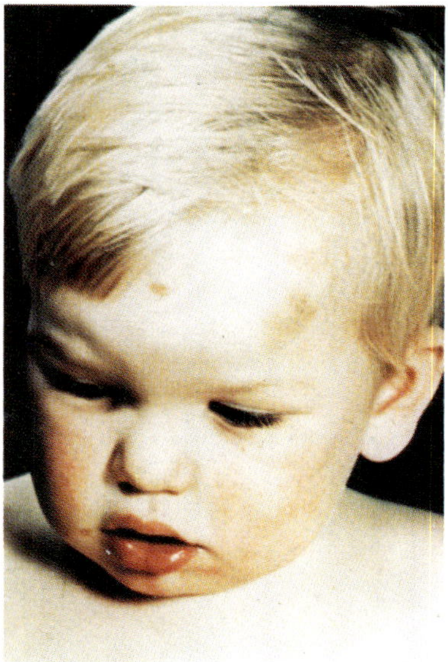

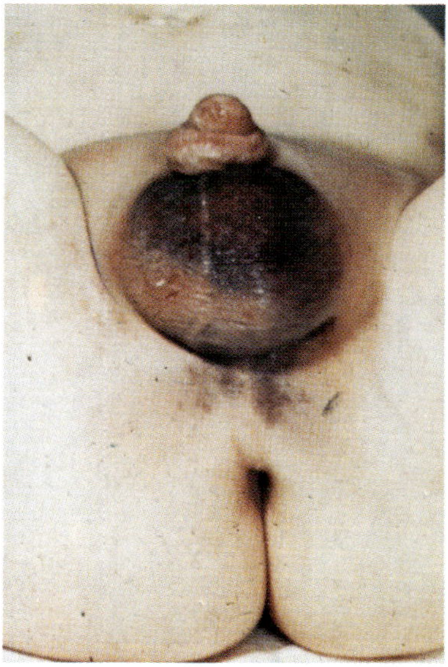

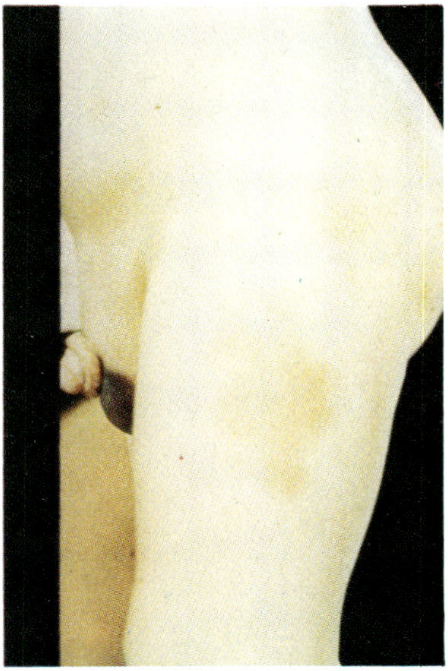

Plate 7. Male aged 2 years admitted with facial bruising attributed by the mother to falling from a chair

Plate 8. Same child as in Plate 7 showing bruising to the scrotum and perineum attributed by the mother to a door accidentally slamming on him

Plate 9. Same child as in Plates 6 and 7 showing bruising to the lateral aspect of the left thigh and buttock, also attributed to a door slamming on him. Later discovered that bruising resulted from periodic kickings from the boy's mother

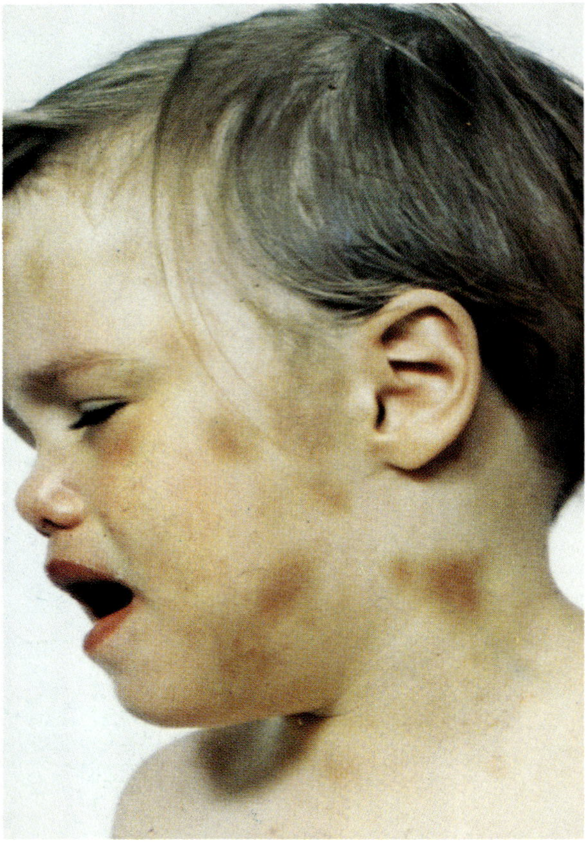

Plate 10. Female aged 3 years admitted with multiple bruising to the face. The child had been slapped by the mother because she had refused her food

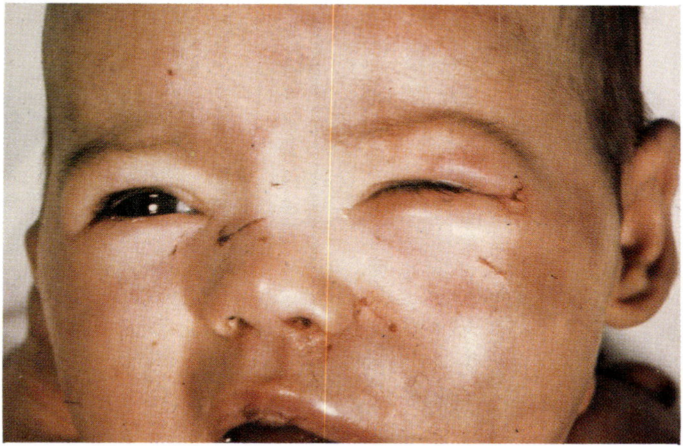

Plate 11. Female aged 18 months admitted with scalds and abrasions to the face, attributed by the parents to 'accidental spilling of a cup of tea'

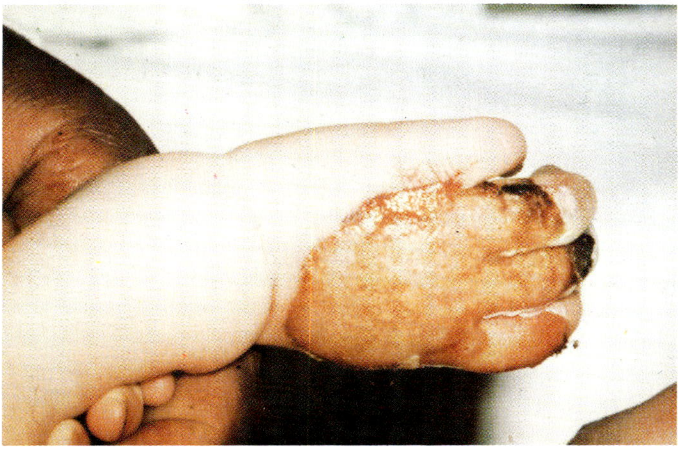

Plate 12. Same child as in Plate 11 showing a burn to the left hand caused, according to the parents, by the child 'placing its hand against a hot electric light bulb'. This burn had been treated at another hospital 1 week previously. Skeletal survey revealed an old fracture of the left wrist

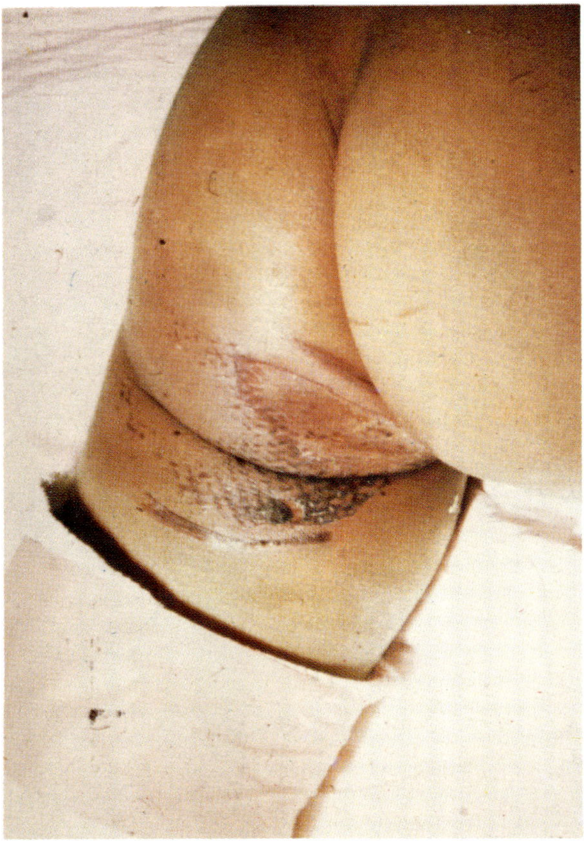

Plate 13. Indian female aged 3 years showing a burn to the buttock and perineum, attributed by the parents to scalding from a pot of hot water placed under the child in an attempt to overcome her constipation. Later discovered to be the result of deliberately placing the child on a hot paraffin heater. Skeletal survey revealed a fractured left tibia and fibula

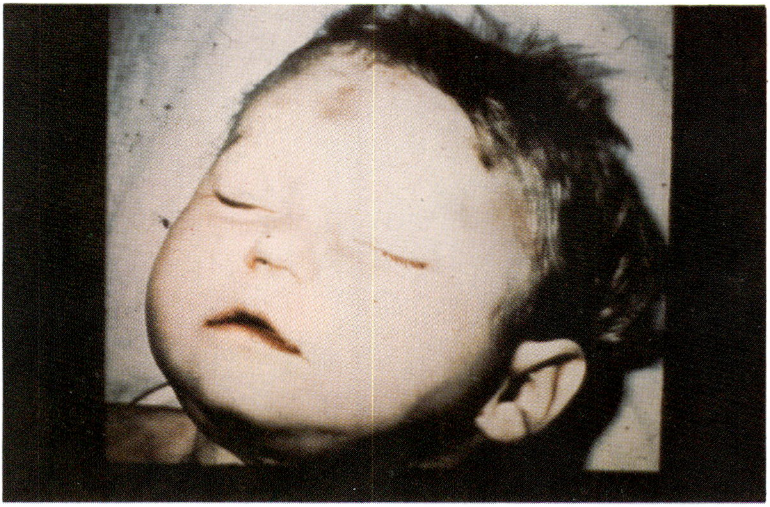

Plate 14. Male aged 27 months showing bruising of the forehead and temples. Mother provided the history that the child 'had fallen over'. The child was drowsy, but was not admitted to hospital and a skull x-ray was not taken. Several hours later the mother returned to the same casualty department| and offered the explanation that her boyfriend had beaten the boy. The child was dead on arrival

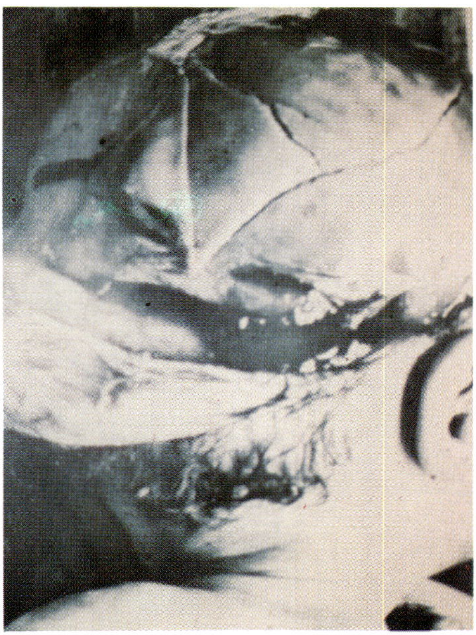

Plate 15. Same child as in Plate 14, showing an extensively depressed skull fracture. The child also had a subdural and cerebral haemorrhage, caused when the mother's boyfriend swung the child against a brick wall

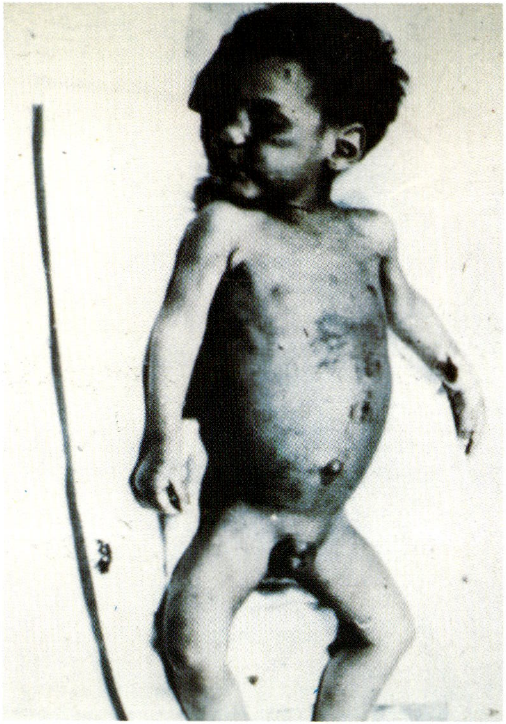

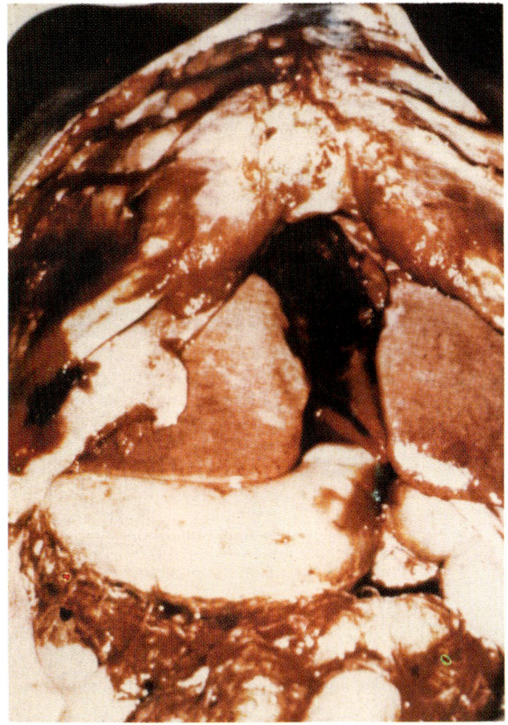

Plates 16 and 17. Dead child showing extensive body bruising. Plate 17 shows the liver split in two – a result of a blow/blows to the abdomen by the boy's father

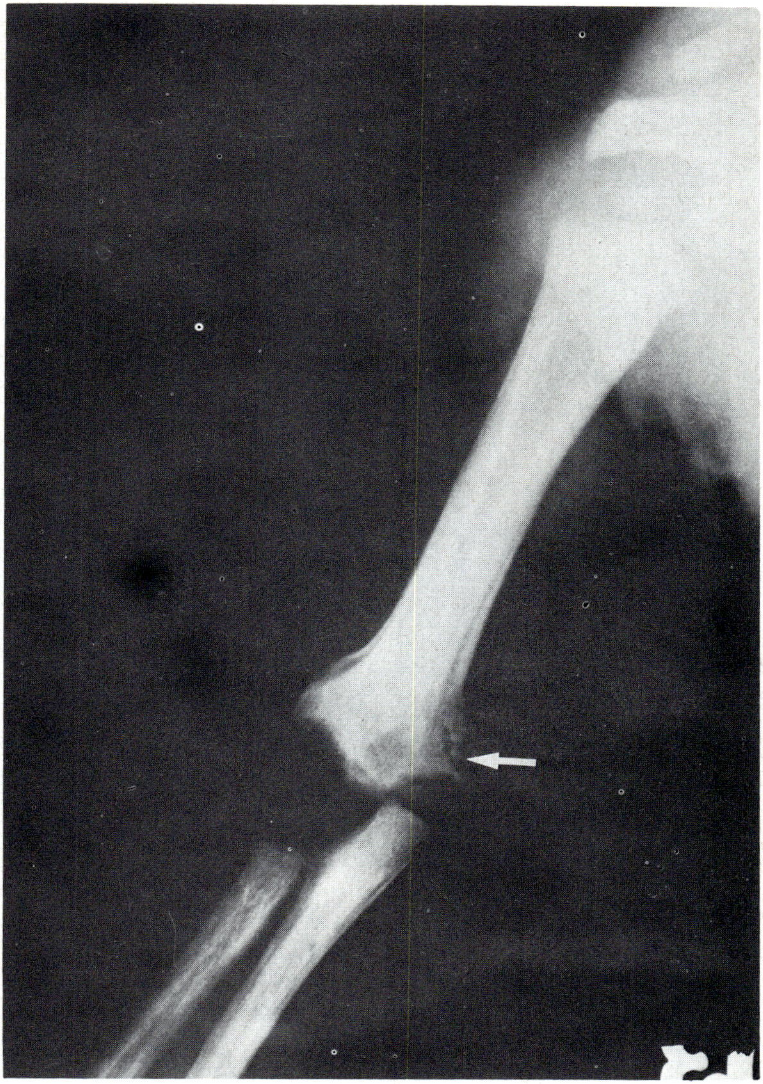

Figure 23. The right humerus and elbow shows appearances similar to Figure 22 at the lower humeral metaphyseal region with a more absorbed periosteal reaction indicating that trauma has occurred earlier. The peripheral new bone along the radial and ulna shafts has almost absorbed leaving uniformly thickened bones

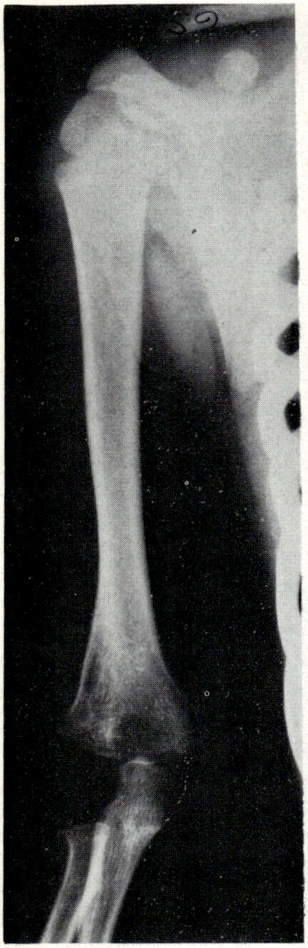

Figure 24

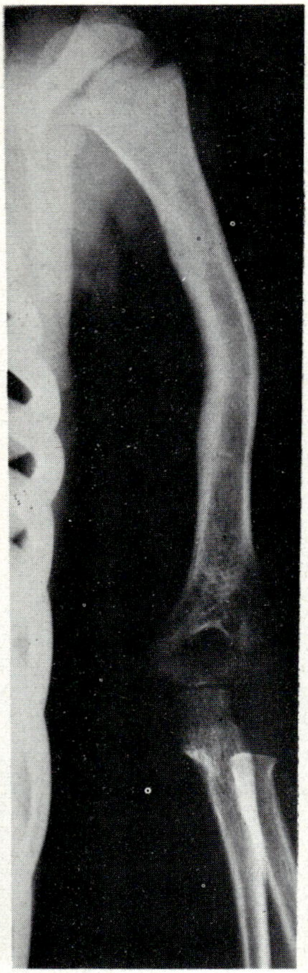

Figure 25

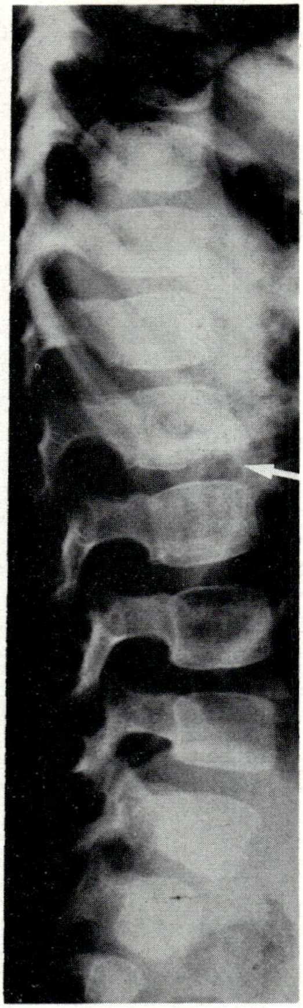

Figure 26

Figure 24. Normal right humerus for comparison with Figure 25

Figure 25. Left humerus, showing that the cortex of the midshaft is of uneven thickness and bowed in different directions at several levels, indicating multiple sites of fractures in the past

Figure 26. Vertebral Column: The body of L2 is widened and irregular adjacent to its lower disc margin suggesting recurrent disruption at the bone forming cartilage – an unusual injury

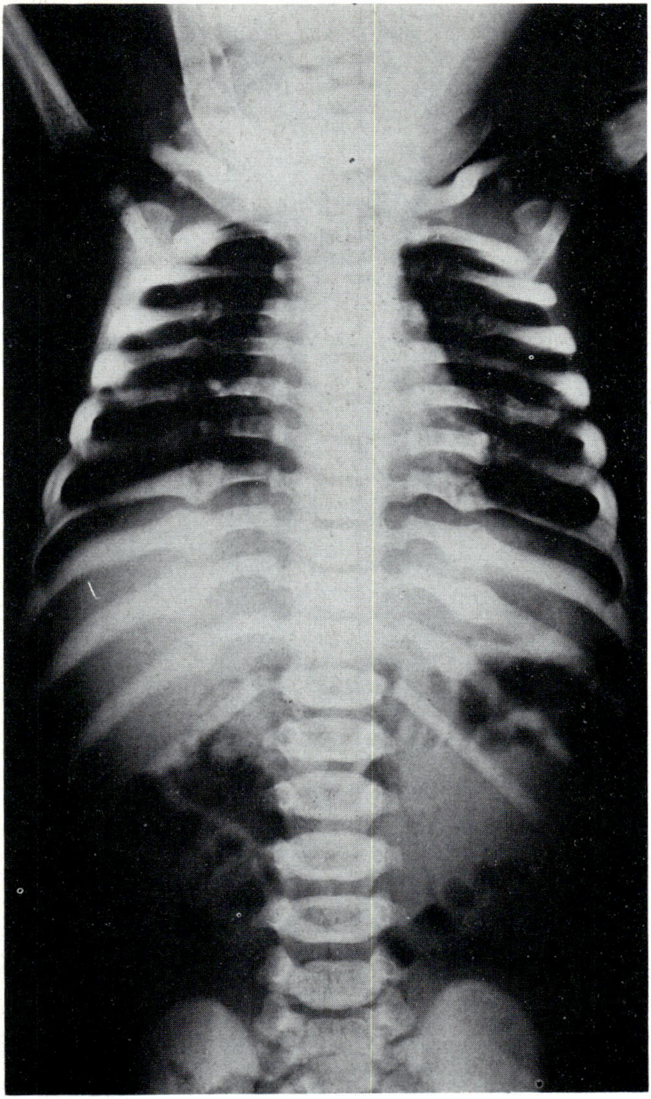

Figure 27. Thoracic Cage: Fractures crossing the posterior parts of nearly all the ribs are well seen because they have widened and are surrounded by abundant callus. These features suggest that healing has been hindered by recurrent trauma or undernutrition

PART III

PSYCHIATRIC, PSYCHOLOGICAL AND SOCIAL CHARACTERISTICS OF THE PARENTS

Chapter 13

Psychiatric Characteristics

PERSONALITY CHARACTERISTICS

AGE OF PARENTS

The mean age of the index mothers was 23.5 years, a high proportion of whom were aged 21 at the time of the child's injury (*see Figure 28*). The mean age of index fathers was 27.0 years, and their age distribution was similar to the mothers (*see Figure 29*).

SOCIAL CLASS

It was found the index group cases were of significantly lower social class than the controls ($p < 0.001$). Among the index parents none came from social class I and only three were from social class II (*see* Table 8).

TABLE 8
Social Class Distribution among Index and Control Groups

	I	II (*Non-manual*)	III	IV	V (*Manual*)
Index group (%)	0 (0)	3 (2.5)	26 (22.0)	56 (47.5)	33 (28.0)
Control group (%)	5 (9.6)	4 (7.7)	26 (50.0)	14 (26.9)	3 (5.8)

χ^2 with 1 d.f. = 26.29, $p < 0.001$

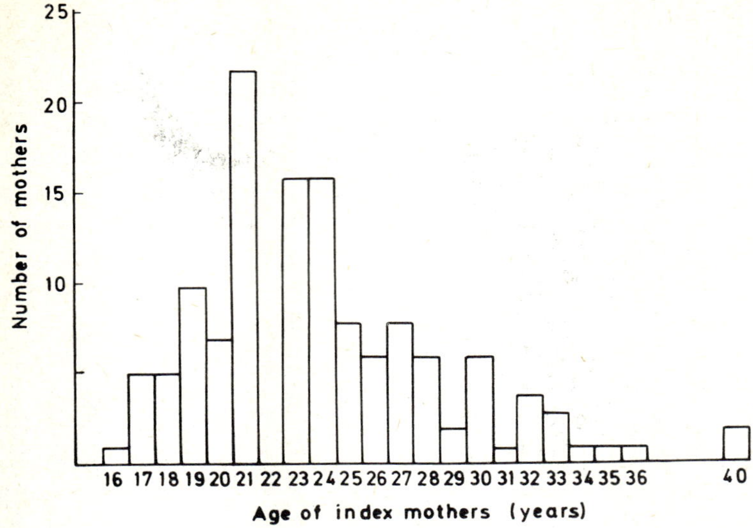

Figure 28. Age of index mothers

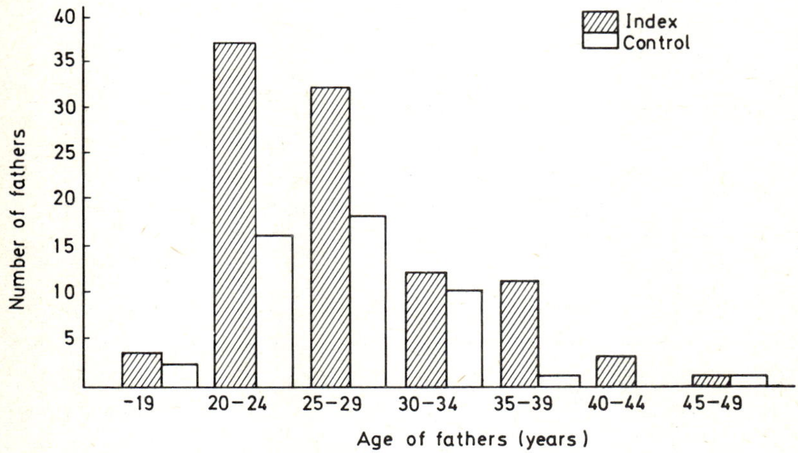

Figure 29. Age of index fathers

PERSONALITY

Ninety-five of the 125 mothers (76 per cent) and 57 of the 89 fathers (64 per cent) in the index group had an abnormal personality. Compared with the controls this amount of abnormality was highly significant ($p < 0.001$) (*see* Table 9). Adjustments for social class did not alter the significance levels of these findings.

SEVERITY OF PERSONALITY DISORDER

Seventy-eight mothers (62.4 per cent) had personality disorders of mild or moderate severity compared with the controls. This was a significant finding (for 1 d.f. and $\chi^2 = 45.32$; $p < 0.001$). Twenty-four fathers (27 per cent) had mild or moderately severe personality disorders and this also was significantly different from the controls (for 1 d.f. and $\chi^2 = 5.63$; $p < 0.05$). Seventeen mothers (13.6 per cent) and 33 fathers (37.1 per cent) in the index group had severe personality or psychopathic disorders.

TABLE 9
Comparison of Personality Findings in Parents in Both Groups

	Normal		*Abnormal*		
	No.	*Per cent*	*No.*	*Per cent*	
Index mothers	30	24.0	95	76.0	*
Control mothers	44	86.3	7	13.7	
Index fathers	32	36.0	57	64.0	†
Control fathers	21	87.5	3	12.5	

* $\chi^2 = 55.12$; d.f. = 1; $p < 0.001$
† $\chi^2 = 18.15$; d.f. = 1; $p < 0.001$

None of the controls were psychopathic. Nine mothers (7.2 per cent) and 29 fathers (32.6 per cent) were aggressive psychopaths. Eight mothers (6.4 per cent) and 4 fathers (4.5 per cent) were inadequate psychopaths. Alcoholism and drug dependence was not a feature among the index cases or controls.

NEUROSIS

Among the index group 60 mothers (48 per cent) and 9 fathers (10.1 per cent) were neurotic. Compared with the controls neurosis was a significant finding ($p < 0.001$) among index mothers only (*see* Table 10).

TABLE 10
Comparison of Neurosis Findings in
Index and Control Mothers

	Non-neurotic		*Neurotic*	
	No.	*Per cent*	*No.*	*Per cent*
Index group	65	52.0	60	48.0
Control group	46	90.2	5	9.8

$\chi^2 = 12.08$; d.f. = 1; $p < 0.001$

Of the index mothers 34 (27.2 per cent) showed mixed neurotic symptomatology, 21 (16.8 per cent) were depressed, 2 (1.6 per cent) showed anxiety reactions and 2 (1.6 per cent) had hysterical reactions. One subject (0.8 per cent) was agoraphobic. Of the control mothers 5 (9.8 per cent) showed a mixed neurotic picture. One index mother had anorexia nervosa. Her case has been described in detail elsewhere (Smith and Hanson, 1972).

GENERAL HEALTH QUESTIONNAIRE

Mean scores for index mothers were 19.2 compared with 7.2 for controls ($t = 5.27$; $p < 0.001$). Mean scores for index fathers were 11.0 compared with 6.1 for controls ($t = 1.93$; $p = 0.57$). This finding supports the validity of clinical diagnosis of neurosis found among index mothers (mentioned above).

EYSENCK PERSONALITY INVENTORY

Mothers

High scoring (20 +) on the neuroticism (N) scale of the inventory was significantly more characteristic of index than control mothers (for 1 d.f. and $\chi^2 = 4.69$; $p < 0.05$). On the Extraversion scale the mean scores for index and controls were 13.3 and 13.8 respectively. The difference was not significant. Mean Lie scores were 3.2 for index and 2.3 for controls ($t = 3.51$; $p < 0.001$). *Figure 30* compares Neuroticism scores of index and control mothers with the normal female population (Eysenck and Eysenck, 1964). Mean Neuroticism scores were 14.4 for index and 12.9 for controls ($t = 1.92$; $p < 0.57$). Excluding those who scored 4 + on the Lie scale (48 index and 10

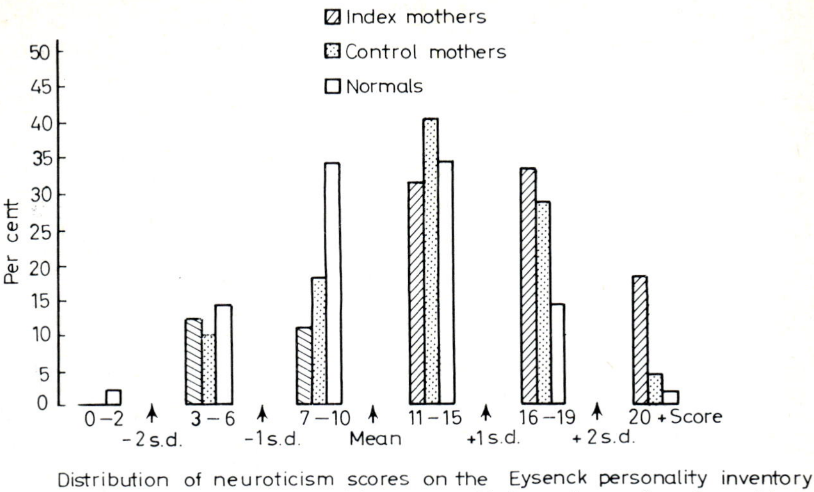

Figure 30. Comparison of Neuroticism scores of index and control mothers with the normal female population

controls) the means were 14.9 and 13.0 respectively and this difference was statistically significant ($t = 2.04$; $p < 0.05$).

Fathers

On the Extraversion scale the mean scores for index and control fathers were 15.1 and 16.1 respectively. Mean Lie scores were 2.5 for index and 2.0 for controls. Mean Neuroticism scores were 9.6 for index and 9.9 for the controls. After excluding those who scored 4 + on the Lie scale (20 index and 3 controls) the means were 10.0 and 9.2 respectively. None of these differences were statistically significant.

HOSTILITY AND DIRECTION OF HOSTILITY QUESTIONNAIRE

Mothers

The mean Total Hostility scores were 22.8 for index and 17.6 for controls ($t = 4.01$; $p < 0.001$). *Figure 31* shows the mean scores on

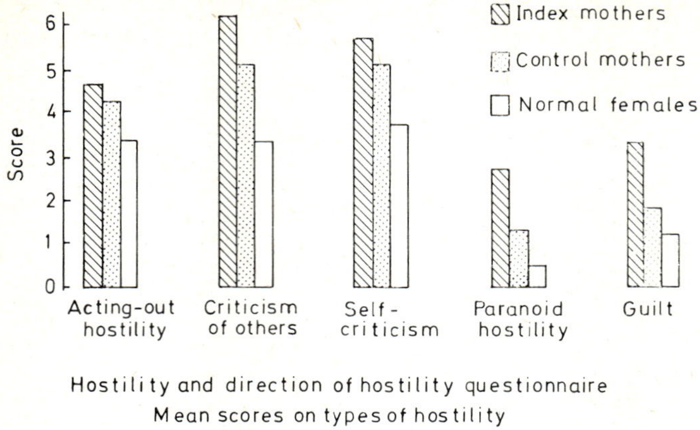

Figure 31. Comparison of mean Hostility scores (H.D.H.Q.) among index and control mothers and normal females

the various types of hostility for index and control mothers and compares them with normal females (Caine *et al.*, 1967). Significant differences were found on Criticism of Others ($t = 2.61$; $p < 0.01$); Paranoid Hostility ($t = 4.75$; $p < 0.001$) and Guilt ($t = 4.63$; $p < 0.001$). When those with 4+ Lie scores on the Eysenck Personality Inventory were excluded from the index sample, index mothers scored higher than controls on Acting Out Hostility (means 5.1 and 4.3 respectively, $p < 0.05$), Criticism of Others (means 6.1 and 5.1 respectively, $p < 0.05$) and Self-Criticism (means 5.9 and 5.1 respectively, $p < 0.05$). The Direction of Hostility score was not found to be a useful discriminator between index and controls.

Fathers

The mean Total Hostility scores were 18.6 for index and 16.9 for controls (difference not significant). *Figure 32* shows the mean scores on the various types of hostility for index and control fathers and compares them with normal males (Caine, Foulds and Hope, 1967). Among the types of hostility the only significant difference found between index and control fathers was on Guilt. The means were 2.2 and 1.4 respectively ($t = 2.06$; $p < 0.05$). Differences on Paranoid Hostility approached significance.

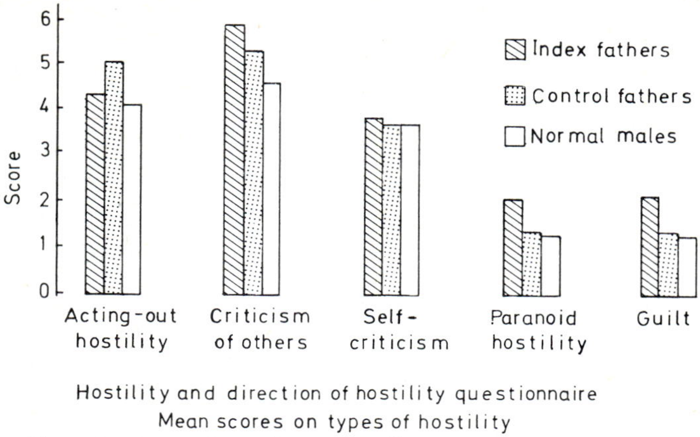

Figure 32. Comparison of mean Hostility scores (H.D.H.Q.) among index and control fathers and normal males

PSYCHOSIS

Psychotic reactions were observed in 4 mothers (3.2 per cent) and 1 father (1.1 per cent). None of the controls were psychotic. Two mothers were paranoid schizophrenics; one of them killed her two children under the influence of hallucinations. She was found unfit to plead and committed to a special hospital. Two mothers and one father were psychotically depressed. The injuries inflicted on the children by psychotic parents were bizarre.

CRIMINAL RECORDS

Excluding juvenile court appearances among the index group 29.2 per cent of the fathers and 11.2 per cent of the mothers had a criminal record (*see* Table 11). Of the control group none of the mothers and

TABLE 11
Number of Parents with Criminal Records in the Index Group

	Number of criminal records investigated	*Number with criminal records after child abuse incident*	*Total number with criminal records*
Fathers	89	6 (6.7 per cent)	26 (29.2 per cent)
Mothers	125	5 (4.0 per cent)	14 (11.2 per cent)

only two of the fathers had a criminal record. After the child abuse incident subsequent criminal convictions for offences other than child abuse occurred in 6.7 per cent of fathers and 4 per cent of mothers. Twenty-three fathers (25.8 per cent) and 13 mothers (10.4 per cent) in the index group had been convicted for theft or larceny (*see* Table 12). Convictions for violent crimes were recorded in 8 fathers (9.0 per cent) and 1 mother (0.8 per cent). Four of the fathers (4.5 per cent) had convictions for sexual offences including rape. Cruelty and neglect to children were recorded in only 1 mother and 1 father.

TABLE 12
Types of Criminal Offences in Index Group

Criminal offences	*Fathers* (n = *89*)	*Mothers* (n = *125*)
Theft, larceny etc.	23	13
Crimes of violence	8	1
Serious sexual offences	4	0
Cruelty and neglect to children	1	1
Motoring and traffic offences	2	0
Drunk and disorderly	1	1
Breach of probation order	0	1

INTELLIGENCE

The mean I.Q.s (based on the combined subtests) were 80 for index mothers, 95 for controls, 92 for index fathers and 102 for controls. The difference in distribution of I.Q.s between the index and control mothers was highly significant (for 2 d.f. $\chi^2 = 28.61$; $p < 0.001$). Index and control fathers were also different in ability but the differences were not as statistically significant. The distribution of mothers' I.Q.s are shown in *Figure 33.* Nearly half the sample of index mothers were on borderline subnormality or below.

GIBSON SPIRAL MAZE

Mean Time scores were 43.0 sec for index mothers and 37.5 sec for the controls. This difference was significant ($t = 3.57$; $p < 0.001$). Mean Error scores were 20.2 for index mothers and 14.0 for the controls. This difference was also significant ($t = 2.19$; $p < 0.05$). On

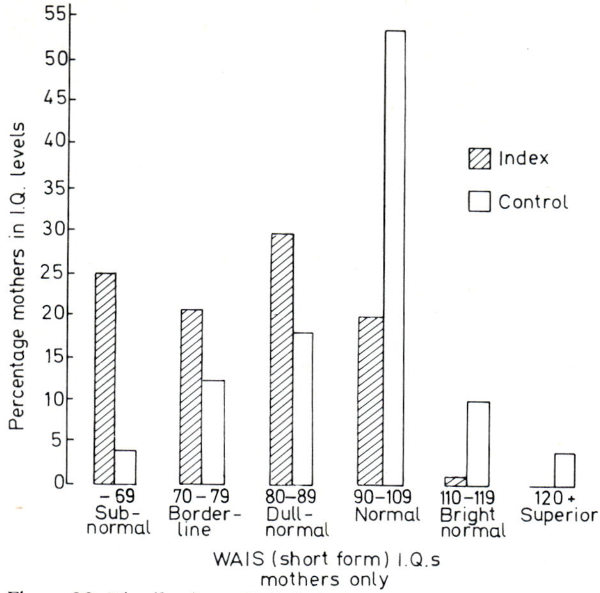

Figure 33. Distribution of I.Q. in index and control mothers (Wechsler Adult Intelligence Scale)

the 'quick and careless' dimension the difference between index and control mothers was not significant. Index mothers were significantly more 'slow and clumsy' than control mothers ($\chi^2 = 12.17$; d.f. = 1; $p < 0.001$).

Index and control fathers did not differ significantly on Time and Error scores.

ELECTROENCEPHALOGRAMS

Eight parents (23 per cent) had demonstrably abnormal EEGs. In the case of the other 27 batterers and 15 of their spouses no EEG abnormality was shown. The one remaining spouse who was known to have epilspsy but was not responsible for baby battering had a characteristically abnormal EEG. No abnormal response to 3 min hyperventilation occurred in any of the subjects.

On further investigation the eight batterers with abnormal EEGs were generally found to be of low intelligence though no lower on

TABLE 13
Performance I.Q. and EEG Findings

Performance I.Q. (WAIS)	*EEG normal*	*EEG abnormal*
Subnormal to borderline	8	1
Dull normal to average	4	5

Males are not included in this table since there was only one with an abnormal EEG.

average than those subjects in whom no EEG abnormality could be shown. Of the women tested those with an abnormal EEG tended to score higher on performance subtests than did those with a normal EEG (*see* Table 13). All eight subjects with abnormal EEGs had a personality disorder without reference to the act of battering (*see* Table 14). They were also found to be persistent batterers – that is, to have battered one child more than once and sometimes more than one of their children.

TABLE 14
Personality Diagnoses and EEG Findings

Personality Diagnosis	*EEG normal*		*EEG abnormal*	
	Male	*Female*	*Male*	*Female*
Personality disorder (mild and moderate severity)	3	9	–	2
Aggressive psychopathy	6	3	1	5

RECOLLECTIONS OF CHILDHOOD

MOTHERS

NEUROTIC SYMPTOMS IN CHILDHOOD

Forty-two index (34 per cent) compared with 2 control mothers (4 per cent) were unhappy in childhood ($\chi^2 = 15.87$; d.f. = 1; $p < 0.001$); Sixty-two index (51 per cent) compared with 4 controls (8 per cent) had 2 or more neurotic symptoms in childhood ($\chi^2 = 26.84$; d.f. = 1; $p < 0.001$). Both these findings remained significant after class control.

The types of individual neurotic symptoms were nail-biting 50 (50 per cent), 'nervous' child 24 (24 per cent), nightmares 10 (10 per cent), thumb-sucking 9 (9 per cent), enuresis 8 (8 per cent), temper tantrums 7 (7 per cent), stammering 6 (6 per cent) and fear of the dark

3 (3 per cent). Other miscellaneous neurotic symptoms were reported by 23 (23 per cent) index mothers. Seventeen (17 per cent) index and none of the controls reported that they were emotionally handicapped as a result of these symptoms.

PHYSICAL HEALTH AND HEAD INJURY

Three index (2 per cent) and 2 controls (4 per cent) had convulsions in childhood. Ten index (8 per cent) had had some degree of physical handicap.

Fifteen index (12 per cent) and 1 control (2 per cent) had suffered serious accidental head injuries, but the difference did not reach statistical significance.

SCHOOL SUCCESS

Forty-one index (34 per cent) and none of the controls regarded themselves as poor scholars ($\chi^2 = 20.64$; d.f. = 1; $p < 0.001$). This finding remained significant after class control. Ten index (8 per cent) and none of the controls had attended special schools because of their emotional or physical handicaps. Forty-three index (35 per cent) compared with 8 controls (16 per cent) were unhappy at school ($\chi^2 = 5.71$; d.f. = 1; $p < 0.05$). This difference became insignificant after adjustments were made for social class.

FAMILY HISTORY OF PSYCHIATRIC ILLNESS

Thirty-three index (27 per cent) compared with 6 controls (12 per cent) had close relatives who had been hospitalized for psychiatric illness ($\chi^2 = 4.08$; d.f. = 1; $p < 0.05$). When social class adjustments were made the contrast became insignificant. Thirty-eight index (31 per cent) compared with 10 control mothers (20 per cent) had relatives who suffered from 'nerves', but the difference was not significant.

INTERPERSONAL RELATIONSHIPS IN CHILD- AND ADULTHOOD

Parents

Forty-three index (36 per cent) and 4 controls (8 per cent) had impaired relationships with their parents ($\chi^2 = 11.93$; d.f. = 1; $p < 0.001$). In childhood the proportions were 39 (32 per cent) and 4 (8 per cent) respectively ($\chi^2 = 9.63$; d.f. = 1; $p < 0.01$). Both these differences remained significant after class control.

Siblings

Twenty-two index (19 per cent) and 1 control (2 per cent) had impaired relationships with their siblings ($\chi^2 = 6.77$; d.f. = 1; $p < 0.01$). In childhood the proportions were 39 (32 per cent) and 4 (8 per cent) respectively ($\chi^2 = 9.63$; d.f. = 1; $p < 0.01$). Both these differences remained significant after class control.

Friends

Fifty-six index (46 per cent) compared with 8 controls (16 per cent) had no friends ($\chi^2 = 12.55$; d.f. = 1; $p < 0.001$). This finding held after class control. In childhood the proportions were 24 (20 per cent) and 10 (20 per cent) respectively and this difference was not significant.

Upbringing

The chief technique of discipline employed by their own mothers was scolding. This was reported by 63 index mothers (57 per cent) and 39 controls (80 per cent). This difference was significant ($\chi^2 = 6.71$; d.f. = 1; $p < 0.01$) and remained so after class control.

Table 15 describes the types of discipline experienced by both index and control mothers during their childhoods. A significant proportion of index mothers described their own mothers and fathers as unreasonable in their discipline. A smaller but nevertheless significant proportion described their parents as harsh and rejecting. The significant differences shown in the table remained after adjusting for social class.

Eighty index mothers (70 per cent) compared with 47 controls (90 per cent) described their own mothers as warm and affectionate ($\chi^2 = 7.42$; d.f. = 1; $p < 0.01$). This finding became insignificant after adjustments were made for social class. Sixty-nine index (73 per cent) compared with 45 controls (88 per cent) described their own fathers as warm and affectionate. This difference did not reach statistical significance.

TABLE 15
Types of Discipline Experienced by Index and Control Mothers in Childhood

Mothers' upbringing by own mother	*Index*		*Control*		*Significance (d.f. = 1)*	
	No.	*Per cent*	*No.*	*Per cent*	χ^2	*p*
Reasonable	65	(55)	50	(100)	30.76*	< 0.001
Strict	26	(22)	0	(0)		
Rejecting	19	(16)	0	(0)	11.99†	< 0.001
Harsh	8	(7)	0	(0)		
Mothers' upbringing by own father						
Reasonable	54	(40)	45	(92)	24.56*	< 0.001
Strict	20	(18)	0	(0)		
Rejecting	18	(16)	3	(6)	9.59†	< 0.01
Harsh	18	(16)	1	(2)		

* Reasonable vs strict, rejecting and harsh
† Reasonable and strict vs rejecting and harsh

FATHERS

HEAD INJURY

Thirty-six index fathers (40 per cent) compared with 3 controls (13 per cent) had suffered serious accidental head injuries ($\chi^2 = 5.36$; d.f. = 1; $p < 0.05$). This difference became insignificant after adjustments were made for social class.

UPBRINGING

Twenty-six index fathers (32 per cent) and none of the controls described their mothers as unreasonable in their discipline ($\chi^2 = 7.69$; d.f. = 1; $p < 0.01$). This difference remained significant after class control. Thirty-five index (44 per cent) and 2 controls (10 per cent) described their fathers as unreasonable ($\chi^2 = 6.97$; d.f. = 1; $p < 0.01$). This difference also remained significant after class control.

On all other recollections of childhood index fathers did not differ significantly from the controls.

Chapter 14

Social Characteristics

SOCIAL ASPECTS OF THE FAMILIES

MARITAL STATUS

Of the index mothers 36 (29 per cent) were unmarried, compared with 3 control mothers (6 per cent) ($\chi^2 = 10.19$; d.f. = 1; $p < 0.01$). In 44 index (35 per cent) compared with 2 control cases (4 per cent), the biological father was absent ($\chi^2 = 17.17$; d.f. = 1; $p < 0.001$). Table 16 shows the situation at time of interview.

TABLE 16
Family Situation of Index Mothers (n = 124)

Status	*No.*	*Per cent*
Single and living alone	19	15
Single and cohabiting	4	3
Separated and living alone	6	5
Separated and cohabiting	7	6
Separated and married	7	6
Total	43	35

More than half the index mothers (54 per cent) had given birth to their first child before the age of 20 compared with 10.6 per cent in the population at large (Registrar General, 1973, Part 2). Twelve index (15 per cent) compared with none of the controls ($\chi^2 = 6.62$; d.f. = 1; $p < 0.01$) knew each other for less than 6 months before marriage. Among the index group 36 mothers (30 per cent) and 11 fathers (13 per cent) described their marriage or liaison as unsatisfactory. No control parent reported this. This was significant ($\chi^2 = 17.43$; d.f. = 1; $p < 0.001$) for index mothers only. All these findings held after controlling for class.

PRE-MARITAL CONCEPTION AND ILLEGITIMACY

Eighty-seven index mothers (71 per cent) compared with 17 controls (33 per cent) had conceived pre-maritally ($\chi^2 = 19.44$; d.f. = 1; $p < 0.001$). Forty-five battered children (36 per cent) compared with 3 controls (6 per cent) were illegitimate ($\chi^2 = 15.48$; d.f. = 1; $p < 0.001$). Table 17 shows the occurrence of pre-marital conception and illegitimacy broken down by age and compares both with national norms (Registrar General, 1973, Part 2). In every age group index mothers have pre-marital pregnancies and illegitimate babies much more frequently. Social class adjustments did not affect these findings.

TABLE 17
Pre-Marital Conception and Illegitimacy Rates of Index and Census Mothers by Age

Mother's age	*Pre-marital pregnancy (per cent)*		*Illegitimacy (per cent)*	
	Index	*Census*	*Index*	*Census*
15–19	94.1	69.7	33.3	25.8
20–24	48.2	20.6	25.9	7.7
25–29	52.9	7.1	50.0	4.6
30–34	25.0	6.4	50.0	5.5

ATTITUDE TO PREGNANCY AND ABORTION

Twenty three index mothers (20 per cent) compared with 3 controls (6 per cent) were displeased ($\chi^2 = 4.32$; d.f. = 1; $p < 0.05$). Fifteen index (13 per cent) compared with none of the controls claimed that their partners were displeased over the pregnancy ($\chi^2 = 6.14$; d.f. = 1; $p < 0.05$). This finding was not significant, when class was taken into account. Fifty-seven index (49 per cent) compared with 19 control mothers (37 per cent) had reservations about the pregnancy but this was not a significant finding. Fifteen index mothers (12 per cent) and only 1 control mother (2 per cent) had considered an abortion during the relevant pregnancy, but this difference was not significant (*see* Table 18).

TABLE 18
Use of and Attitude towards Contraception and Abortion Among Index and Control Mothers

	Index mothers		*Control mothers*		*Significance (d.f. = 1)*	
	No.	*Per cent*	*No.*	*Per cent*	χ^2	*p*
Using contraceptives	42/121	(35)	13/51	(26)	1.01	N.S.
Not using contraceptives and negative attitude	43/79	(54)	8/38	(21)	10.32	< 0.01
Abortion considered	15/121	(12)	1/51	(2)	3.48	N.S.

CONTRACEPTION

Forty-two index mothers (35 per cent) were using contraceptives but those who did not expressed a negative attitude significantly more often than did the control mothers towards the future taking of contraceptives. This remained true after adjustments for social class.

FAMILY SIZE

The mean number of children in the index families was 2.3 and for controls 2.0 ($\chi^2 = 6.62$; d.f. = 1; $p < 0.01$). Forty-three battered babies (32 per cent) were first-born and only children in the family and 91 (68 per cent) were second or subsequent born children. When family size is taken into account, battered babies were observed to be randomly distributed among the different birth orders (*see* Table 19). In families of two children the observed proportion of second-born was higher than expected ($\chi^2 = 5.76$; d.f. = 1; $p < 0.05$). For the controls it was also the younger child who was admitted to hospital.

PARENTS' FAMILY SIZE OF ORIGIN

The parents' mean family size of origin was 5.6 for index mothers, 4.3 for controls, 4.7 for index fathers and 5.3 for controls (statistically not significant, as the apparently large differences are due to a few very large families).

TABLE 19
Position in Family of Index and Control Children

Family Size	Index Child 1	2	3	4	5	6	7	8	Family Size	Control child 1	2	3	4	5	6	7	8
1	43								1	28							
2	13	37							2	0	11						
3	1	6	10						3	0	1	6					
4	0	1	6	3					4	0	0	1	3				
5	0	3	3	2	4				5	0	0	0	0	0			
6	0	0	0	0	0	2			6	0	0	0	0	0			
7	0	0	0	0	0	0	0		7	0	0	0	0	0	0	1	
8	0	0	0	0	0	0	0	0	8	0	0	0	0	0	0	0	1
Totals	57	47	19	5	4	2	0	0		28	12	7	3	0	0	1	1

FAMILY DISHARMONY

Fifteen index mothers (13 per cent) had low opinions of their partners as compared with none of the controls ($\chi^2 = 5.76$; d.f. = 1; $p < 0.05$). Seventeen (15 per cent) admitted that their partners rejected the child as compared with none of the controls. ($\chi^2 = 5.87$; d.f. = 1; $p < 0.05$). Thirty-one index (27 per cent) as compared with 3 control mothers (6 per cent) reported that they did not participate in child-rearing discussions ($\chi^2 = 19.39$; d.f. = 1; $p < 0.001$). Rejection and non-participation remained significant after class control. Forty-seven (41 per cent) reported disagreement over child rearing ($\chi^2 = 19.39$; d.f. = 1; $p < 0.001$) but this particular contrast disappeared when social class was held constant.

On direct questioning about strained relationships within the family a smaller proportion of index 79 (72 per cent), than controls parents 44 (92 per cent), admitted marriage problems ($\chi^2 = 6.53$; d.f. = 1; $p < 0.05$) and this held after adjustments for social class. Twenty-one index (18 per cent) and one control mother (2 per cent) reported that it was they who took the important family decisions ($\chi^2 = 6.81$; d.f. = 1; $p < 0.01$), and this held after adjustments for social class. Twenty-three index mothers (22 per cent) as compared with 5 controls (10 per cent) reported quarrels not long before their child's admission to hospital (difference not significant).

ETHNIC CHARACTERISTICS

One hundred and two index cases (76 per cent) were White, 19 were West Indian (14 per cent) and 13 were Asian (10 per cent).

Table 20 shows that three characteristics differentiated the West Indians from the rest of the White index sample. These were absence of biological father, frequent use of physical punishment and rare contact with parents. Biological fathers were absent in only two Asian homes (17 per cent). When compared with the White sample the difference was not significant. Nine of the Asians (90 per cent) had rare contact with their parents and when compared with the White sample this was a significant difference ($\chi^2 = 8.09$; d.f. = 1; $p < 0.01$).

TABLE 20
Characteristics of West Indian Group.
Index Cases Only

	West Indian		*White*		*Significance (d.f. = 1)*	
	No.	*Per cent*	*No.*	*Per cent*	χ^2	p
Biological father absent	17/19	(90)	26/94	(28)	23.06	< 0.001
Rare contact with parents	13/19	(68)	35/93	(38)	4.91	< 0.05
Frequent use of physical punishment	14/19	(74)	42/88	(48)	3.24	N.S.

RELIGION

Among the index mothers 71 were Church of England (57 per cent), 23 were Roman Catholic (18 per cent), 15 Nonconformist (12 per cent), 11 (9 per cent) belonged to various Asian religions (2 Sikhs, 2 Hindus, 4 Moslems and 3 unidentified). There were no Jewish mothers, and 5 (4 per cent) declared that they had no religion. Among the index fathers 44 were Church of England (51 per cent), 20 were Roman Catholic (23 per cent), 2 Nonconformist (2 per cent), 13 belonged to Asian religions (3 Sikhs, 2 Hindus, 5 Moslem and 3 unidentified). There were no Jewish fathers, and 7 (8 per cent) declared that they had no religion.

Affiliation was nominal for 71 index mothers (58 per cent) and 46 index fathers (61 per cent).

Among the index group 40 mothers (33 per cent) and 19 fathers (26 per cent) reported a personal faith. For the controls the proportions were 21 mothers (40 per cent) and 5 fathers (25 per cent) but when compared with the index group these were not significantly different. Forty-seven index mothers (39 per cent) and 39 index fathers (54 per cent) reported that at least one of their parents had a personal faith. For the controls the proportions were 15 mothers (29 per cent) and 6 fathers (30 per cent) but when compared with the index group these also were not significantly different.

ACCOMMODATION

The various types of accommodation occupied by index and control families are shown in Table 21. Most index families were living in houses, maisonettes, or flats in small blocks. Only 8 index (6 per cent) and 6 control families (12 per cent) were living in tower block flats. Forty-three index (37 per cent), compared with 13 (25 per cent) of the control homes, were rated as being dilapidated (difference not significant). However, 54 index (43 per cent) compared with 8 controls (15 per cent) had homes lacking in one or more essential amenities ($\chi^2 = 11.29$; d.f. = 1; $p < 0.001$) and class control did not affect this result. Twenty-five index (28 per cent) compared with 3 control homes (6 per cent) were rated as dirty and untidy ($\chi^2 = 8.22$; d.f. = 1; $p < 0.01$). Seventy-three index (60 per cent), compared with 16 control parents (31 per cent) had moved house on more than two occasions in the period of 3 years prior to interview ($\chi^2 = 7.0$; d.f. = 1; $p < 0.01$). One hundred and six index (87 per cent) compared with 32 control children (63 per cent) shared a bedroom with another member of the family ($\chi^2 = 11.53$; d.f. = 1; $p < 0.01$). Eighty-seven index (71 per cent) compared with 22 control homes (43 per cent) had cramped sleeping accommodation ($\chi^2 = 11.07$; d.f. = 1; $p < 0.001$). All these findings, except child's possession of his own room, became insignificant when class was held constant.

TABLE 21
Types of Accommodation Occupied by Index and Control Families

	House		*Maisonette or flat in small block*		*Flat in tall block*		*Sharing house*		*Other**		*Total*
	No.	*Per cent*	*No.*	*Per cent*	*No.*	*Per cent*	*No.*	*Per cent*	*No.*	*Per cent*	
Index	46	(37)	24	(19)	8	(6)	18	(14)	29	(23)	125
Control	24	(46)	9	(17)	6	(12)	7	(14)	6	(12)	52

* Other includes room in multi-occupied house, lodgings or half-way house.

SOCIAL ISOLATION

A sizeable proportion of index mothers reported having infrequent or no contact with their parents, relatives, neighbours or friends (*see* Table 22). Fifty-three (54 per cent) as compared with 16 control mothers (31 per cent) described themselves as lonely ($\chi^2 = 6.80$; d.f. = 1; $p < 0.01$). Thirty-nine index (32 per cent) compared with 5 (10 per cent) control mothers had no social activities ($\chi^2 = 8.65$; d.f. = 1; $p < 0.01$). Fifty-seven index (49 per cent) compared with 13 controls (26 per cent) reported that they had no opportunities of having a break from the child ($\chi^2 = 7.10$; d.f. = 1; $p < 0.01$). When the social class distribution of the two samples was held constant, loneliness and contact with neighbours and friends became insignificant, but on other measures the contrast remained. Boredom was reported by slightly though not significantly more control than index mothers, 29 (57 per cent) as against 51 (44 per cent).

TABLE 22
Indices of Social Isolation Among Index and Control Mothers

	Index		*Control*		*Significance (d.f. = 1)*	
	No.	*Per cent*	*No.*	*Per cent*	χ^2	*p*
Rare contact with parents	57/122	(47)	12/52	(23)	7.56	< 0.01
Rare contact with relatives	60/122	(49)	9/52	(17)	14.17	< 0.001
Rare contact with neighbours	62/121	(51)	17/52	(33)	4.32	< 0.05
Rare contact with friends	68/122	(56)	15/52	(29)	9.52	< 0.01

Only 3 index (4 per cent) and 2 control fathers (10 per cent) reported having no social activities. This contrasts sharply with the marked difference between index and control mothers ($\chi^2 = 8.19$; d.f. = 1; $p < 0.01$). The difference between index mothers and index fathers is also highly significant ($\chi^2 = 18.22$; d.f. = 1; $p < 0.001$) in this same respect.

Of those index mothers who rarely saw their parents, 25 (81 per cent) said they had an unhappy childhood, as compared with 15 (52 per cent) of those who saw their parents frequently ($\chi^2 = 4.42$; d.f. = 1; $p < 0.05$).

INCOME

The average weekly income of index fathers was £21.50 with a range of £8–40 and a median bracket of £21–25. For the controls the mean was £31.00 (*see Figure 34*). Forty-nine index fathers (71 per cent) compared with 9 controls (41 per cent) earned less than £25 per week ($\chi^2 = 5.29$; d.f. = 1; $p < 0.05$). Twenty-two index fathers (31 per cent) regarded their income as 'inadequate', but the differences were not significant when compared with 7 controls (35 per cent).

As previously mentioned index fathers were predominantly manual workers, whereas the control fathers were distributed among the different occupational levels (*see* Table 8). In 1972 the average weekly earnings for manual workers (aged 21–65 years) for Great Britain was £30.90 and for all workers it was £37.00 (Social Trends, 1972). Though both index and control fathers earned less than the national average, this is a reflection of their lower age group (17–46 years). However, when their mean earnings are related to their respective national class populations the disparity is only £3.40 greater, for control than index fathers. Furthermore, when social class is held constant there is no longer a significant contrast between the two groups.

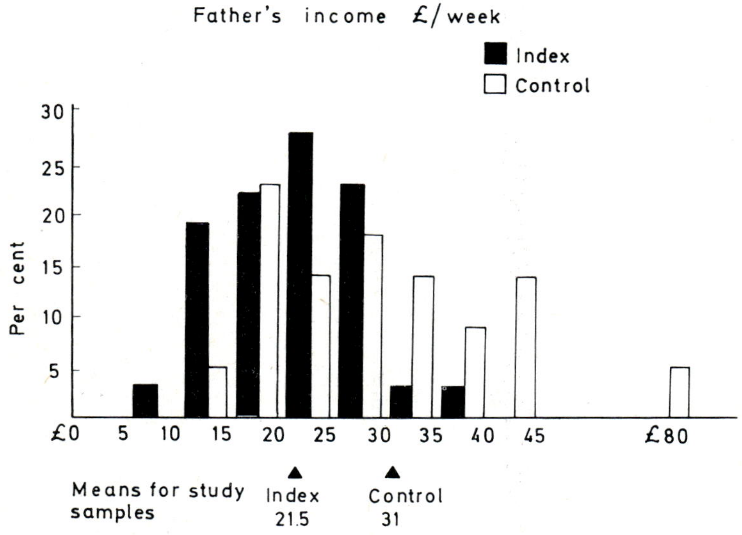

Figure 34. Income of index and control fathers

MOTHERS' ASSESSMENT OF ALLOWANCE AND FOOD EXPENDITURE

Forty-four index (26 per cent) compared with 9 control mothers (18 per cent), regarded their housekeeping allowance as inadequate ($\chi^2 = 5.05$; d.f. = 1; $p < 0.05$). Sixty index (54 per cent) spent less than £2 per head on food per week, compared with 14 control mothers (28 per cent). This difference was significant ($\chi^2 = 8.92$; d.f. = 1; $p < 0.01$) but not after social class had been taken into account.

UNEMPLOYMENT AND STABILITY OF EMPLOYMENT

Fifteen of the index fathers (14 per cent) were unemployed at the time of the battering incident. Seven of the control fathers (13 per cent) were unemployed (difference was not significant). Slightly more, though not significantly more, index than control fathers had changed their jobs on more than five occasions 55 (64 per cent) as against 10 (42 per cent).

DISSATISFACTION

Thirty-two index (26 per cent) compared with two control mothers (4 per cent), reported that they were generally dissatisfied with their total situation ($\chi^2 = 10.24$; d.f. = 1; $p < 0.01$), and this result held after social class control. Thirteen (20 per cent) index compared with none of the control fathers described themselves as being generally dissatisfied.

WORRIES

Ninety-three index (74 per cent), compared with 25 control mothers (48 per cent), reported that they had 2 or more significant worries ($\chi^2 = 7.79$; d.f. = 1; $p < 0.01$). The most frequent worries described were health of others 70 (56 per cent), money 70 (56 per cent), housing 62 (49 per cent), domestic friction 34 (27 per cent), unemployment 33 (26 per cent), own health 31 (25 per cent) and marital status 20 (25 per cent). The rank order was the same for the controls, but the proportion having money and housing problems were lower. Domestic friction, marital status and unemployment were seldom mentioned by the control mothers.

Fifty index (70 per cent) and 8 controls (40 per cent) reported two or more significant worries ($\chi^2 = 5.9$; d.f. = 1; $p < 0.05$). Among the index fathers the worries described were approximately in the same rank order as the index mothers.

The proportion of index parents having worries was no higher than for the control sample when equated for social class.

Chapter 15

Child-rearing Practices and Difficulties Experienced with the Child

CHILD-REARING PRACTICES

MOTHERS

DEMANDS UPON THE CHILD

Crying

Fewer index (68, 59 per cent) than control mothers (41, 79 per cent) allowed the child to cry for a while unless something was obviously wrong ($\chi^2 = 5.59$; d.f. = 1; $p < 0.05$). This difference held after class control. More index (22, 29 per cent) than controls (1, 4 per cent) punished the child for screaming ($\chi^2 = 5.00$; d.f. = 1; $p < 0.05$). Twenty-nine index (28 per cent) compared with 7 controls (29 per cent) isolated the child when it screamed ($\chi^2 = 7.26$; d.f. = 1; $p < 0.01$). When adjusted for social class both these findings became insignificant.

Feeding

Thirty-five index (30 per cent) compared with 13 controls (25 per cent) breast fed their children. Twenty-five index (22 per cent) compared with 9 controls (18 per cent) reported they used rigid feeding schedules. Both these differences were not significant. More index (28, 29 per cent) than controls (3, 6 per cent) became emotionally overinvolved when the child refused food ($\chi^2 = 9.32$; d.f. = 1; $p < 0.01$). The difference remained significant after class control. Emotional over-involvement was significantly associated with mother's neuroticism ($\chi^2 = 5.26$; d.f. = 1; $p < 0.05$).

Cleanliness

Thirty-eight index (36 per cent) compared with 9 control mothers (56 per cent) had commenced potty training before the child was 1 year old; difference not significant. Sixty index (74 per cent) compared with 7 controls (44 per cent) were severe in their training methods ($\chi^2 = 4.42$; d.f. = 1; $p < 0.05$). This difference became insignificant after class control.

Aggression

Fifty-four index (81 per cent) and 10 controls (59 per cent) were not permissive regarding the child's aggressive behaviour (difference not significant). A larger proportion of index (58, 85 per cent) than control mothers (11, 61 per cent) punished aggressive behaviour ($\chi^2 = 3.82$; d.f. = 1; $p < 0.05$). This difference was not significant after controlling for class.

Supervision

A smaller proportion of index (59, 55 per cent) than controls (13, 65 per cent) placed restrictions on the child's access to furniture and other household items (difference not significant). Fewer index (72, 65 per cent) than controls (47, 96 per cent) maintained close surveillance on the child ($\chi^2 = 15.61$; d.f. = 1; $p < 0.001$). This difference held after class control.

Obedience

Eighty-six index (84 per cent) compared with 19 controls (49 per cent) demanded obedience from the child ($\chi^2 = 16.98$; d.f. = 1; $p < 0.001$) A smaller but still significant proportion expected instant obedience – 31 index (30 per cent) compared with 4 controls (10 per cent) – ($\chi^2 = 5.10$; d.f. = 1; $p < 0.05$). The latter finding became insignificant after class control, but moderate demands for obedience held as a significant finding.

METHODS OF CONTROL

Table 23 compares the disciplinary methods used by index and control mothers. Significantly more index than control frequently smacked the child. A smaller but nevertheless significant proportion withheld love as a method of discipline. Good behaviour was materially rewarded more often by index than controls. All these significant differences remained after adjustments were made for social class. Both samples seldom used deprivation of privileges or praise for good behaviour.

TABLE 23
Methods of Controlling their Child (Mothers)

	Index		*Control*		*Significance (d.f. = 1)*	
	No.	*Per cent*	*No.*	*Per cent*	χ^2	*p*
Frequent use of smacking	58/116	(50)	6/47	(13)	17.92	< 0.001
Withholds love	18/106	(17)	1/40	(3)	4.18	< 0.05
Rarely deprives	11/102	(11)	1/27	(4)	0.57	N.S.
Rarely praises	11/113	(10)	1/52	(2)	2.17	N.S.
Gives tangible rewards for good behaviour	53/102	(51)	6/30	(20)	8.08	< 0.01

AFFECTION TOWARDS THE CHILD

Fifty-eight index (49 per cent) compared with 14 control (27 per cent) mothers had little time to play with the child ($\chi^2 = 6.19$; d.f. = 1; $p < 0.05$). This difference was not significant after controlling for class. Fifty-nine index (51 per cent) compared with 7 controls (13 per cent) were not very demonstrative towards the child ($\chi^2 = 18.40$; d.f. = 1; $p < 0.001$). This finding remained significant after class control. Sixty index (50 per cent) compared with 38 controls (73 per cent) enjoyed the child but were glad to get away at times ($\chi^2 = 5.88$; d.f. = 1; $p < 0.05$). This difference remained significant after class control.

FATHERS

More index (24, 37 per cent) than control fathers (2, 10 per cent) reported that they used physical punishment frequently in disciplining their child ($\chi^2 = 4.03$; d.f. = 1; $p < 0.05$). This difference held after

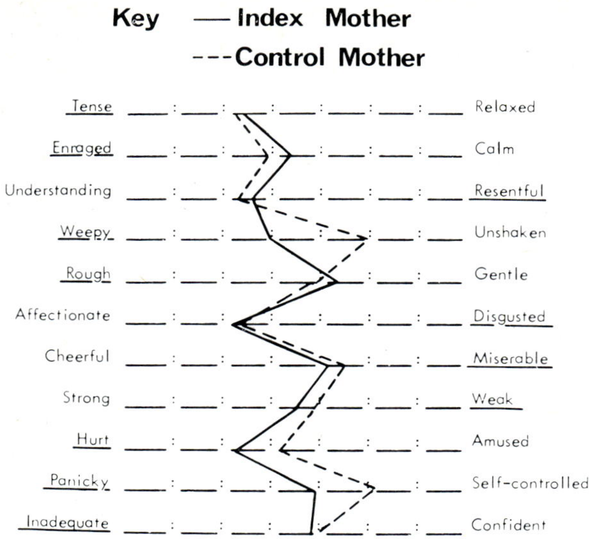

Figure 35. Profile of mean scores on problems with the child. Index and control mothers. (Semantic Differential)

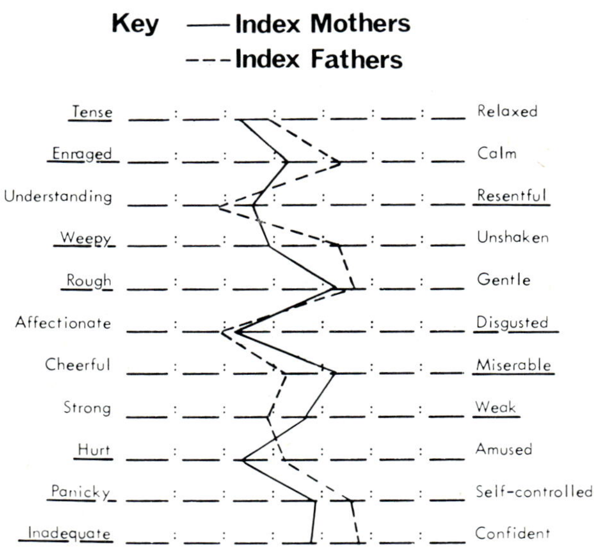

Figure 36. Profile of mean scores on problems with the child. Index mothers and fathers (Semantic Differential)

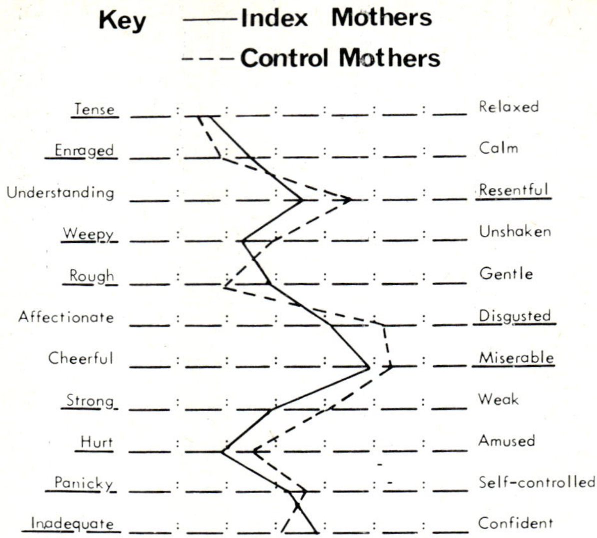

Figure 37. Profile of mean scores on problems with the spouse. Index and control mothers. (Semantic Differential)

social class adjustment. On all other child-rearing methods index fathers did not differ significantly from the controls.

DIFFICULTIES EXPERIENCED WITH THE CHILD

PROBLEMS WITH THE CHILD (DIFFICULT TIMES TEST)

Among the mothers, 39 index (36 per cent) compared with 4 controls (8 per cent) reported that the child's demanding and clinging behaviour was a problem ($\chi^2 = 11.49$; d.f. = 1; $p < 0.001$). Within the index sample this was not related to social class. Screaming in temper was a problem for 17 index (16 per cent) and 8 controls (17 per cent). Messy or destructive behaviour was a problem for 9 index (8 per cent) and 2 controls (4 per cent). Disobedience was a problem for 10 index (8 per cent) and 6 controls (13 per cent). All these differences were not significant.

Failure of the partner to help with caring for the baby was a problem for 22 index (21 per cent) and 2 controls (4 per cent). This difference was significant ($\chi^2 = 5.52$; d.f. = 1; $p < 0.05$). Within the index sample this was not related to social class. Recent quarrels with

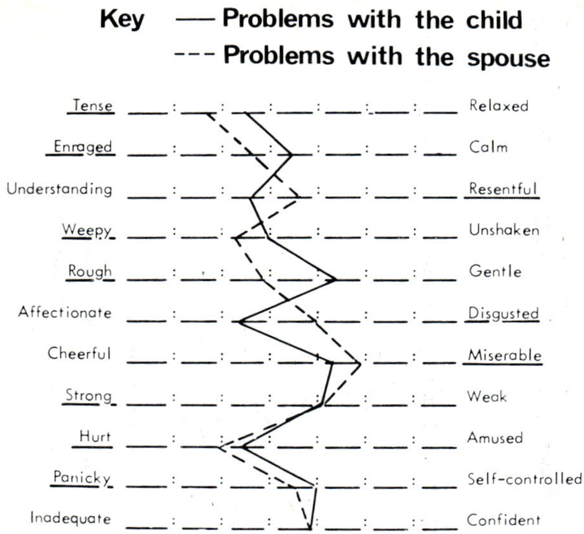

Figure 38. Profile of mean scores comparing child and spouse problems. Index mothers. (Semantic Differential)

the spouse were a problem for 23 index (21 per cent) and 5 controls (10 per cent), but this difference was not significant.

REACTIONS TO PROBLEM BEHAVIOUR (SEMANTIC DIFFERENTIAL)

The means obtained on problems with the child and on problems with the spouse are shown in Table 24.

TABLE 24
Mean Scores on Problems with the Child and Problems with the Spouse (Semantic Differential)

	Problems with the child	*Problems with the spouse*
Index mothers	43.87	52.51
Control mothers	42.32	56.43
Index fathers	36.62	49.14

Control fathers have been excluded from this table because there were too few with these problems to yield reliable results.

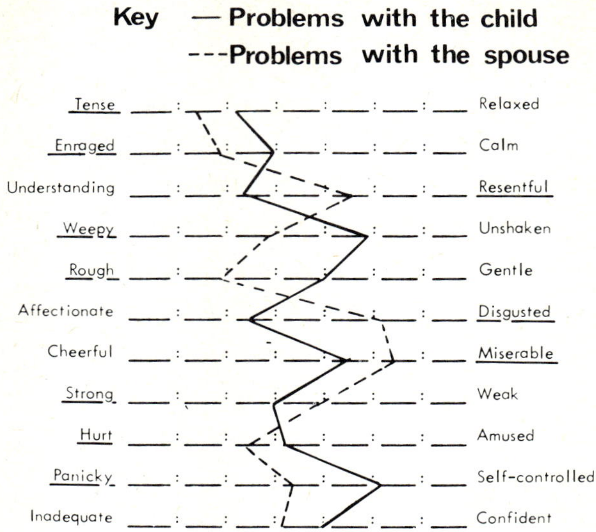

Figure 39. Profile of mean scores comparing child and spouse problems. Control mothers (Semantic Differential)

Tense	___	___	___	___	___	___	___	Relaxed
Enraged	___	___	___	___	___	___	___	Calm
Understanding	___	___	___	___	___	___	___	Resentful
Weepy	___	___	___	___	___	___	___	Unshaken
Rough	___	___	___	___	___	___	___	Gentle
Affectionate	___	___	___	___	___	___	___	Disgusted
Cheerful	___	___	___	___	___	___	___	Miserable
Strong	___	___	___	___	___	___	___	Weak
Hurt	___	___	___	___	___	___	___	Amused
Panicky	___	___	___	___	___	___	___	Self-controlled
Inadequate	___	___	___	___	___	___	___	Confident

Figure 40. Semantic Differential Form

On problems with the child and on problems with the spouse, the difference between index and control mothers, tested by the *t*-test, was not significant. On problems with the child, the difference between index mothers and index fathers was significant ($t = 2.62$; $p < 0.01$). *Figures 35, 36* and *37* illustrate the profiles obtained. These have been compiled by plotting the mean scores on all rating scales listed on the semantic differential form (*see* Appendix B and *Figure 40*) for the following groups: index and control mothers (*see Figure 35*) and index mothers and fathers (*see Figure 36*) on problems with the child, and index and control mothers on problems with the spouse (*see Figure 37*). These figures demonstrate that the profiles comparing index and control mothers are very similar and only differ appreciably on one rating scale; weepy-unshaken. [However, single rating scales are not very reliable (Heise, 1970) and it is advisable to use factor scores based on the combination of at least 4 rating scales, so that this single difference is of little significance.]

By way of contrast, the profiles of index mothers and index fathers are rather dissimilar.

The *t*-test was also applied to the difference between problems with the child and problems with the spouse and this proved to be significant ($t = 3.07$; $p < 0.01$). It was, however, also significant when tested for control mothers ($t = 2.39$, $p < 0.05$). *Figures 38* and *39*, illustrate the differences by means of profiles for each subject-group and problem-group.

Chapter 16

Management Aspects and Characteristics of Identified Perpetrators

MANAGEMENT ASPECTS

DISPOSAL OF THE PARENTS

One hundred and two (81.6 per cent) parents were not prosecuted for battering their child. Of those prosecuted 21 mothers (16.8 per cent) and 10 fathers (11.2 per cent) were sentenced. The method of court disposal and the types of sentence received are shown in Table 25.

TABLE 25
Court Sentencing of Parents

	Mothers (n = *125*)	*Fathers* (n = *89*)
Probation	4	0
Probation with a condition of psychiatric treatment	12	2
Imprisonment	2	7
Discharged	2	0
Special hospital (Broadmoor, Rampton)	3	1
No court appearance	102	79

DISPOSAL OF THE CHILDREN

Table 26 shows the methods of management used by Social Services Departments. Sixty-five battered babies (57.5 per cent) were voluntarily supervised by social workers. Juvenile court proceedings took place in 24 instances (21.2 per cent); care orders being issued in 21 cases (18.6 per cent) and supervision orders in 3 cases (2.6 per cent). Supervision was not arranged in 21 cases (18.6 per cent).

TABLE 26
Management of Battered Children by Social Services Departments

Voluntary supervision	65
Voluntary care	3
No supervision	21
Care order*	21
Supervision order*	3
Not applicable (child died)	21
Total	134

*Juvenile court appearance

THE FOLLOW-UP SURVEY

It was not possible for various reasons to maintain contact with all the index families interviewed. During the course of the study, however, it became apparent that social workers in the field were experiencing certain difficulties in managing these cases. In order to gauge some of these difficulties and assess what possible improvements could be made, the author received the permission of the Assistant Director of Social Services (Birmingham) to circulate a questionnaire to the individual social workers involved. (The questionnaire is available from the author.) The questionnaire was designed only as a preliminary investigation, and though the interpretation of the data presented here should be treated with caution, it does nevertheless, highlight several interesting trends.

The Assistant Director notified each area office that every co-operation should be given in completing the questionnaire. The forms were forwarded directly to the area office that had accepted the case for supervision. Social workers were instructed to return the completed form as soon as possible to the Assistant Director, who then passed them on to the author. The survey covered the period from referral to February 1973.

PRELIMINARY RESULTS

Fifty forms were sent out to the social workers in February 1973. By October 1973, 36 forms had been returned. Eight forms were blank as the Social Services Department had 'no record on these families'. Thus no records could be obtained on 22 (44 per cent) of the 50 cases referred for support to the Social Services Department.

The following preliminary figures are based on the 28 cases (56 per cent) for which records have been obtained. Because the information was incomplete in some cases, percentages are not always based on the same number of cases.

TYPE OF SUPERVISION

At the time of the survey, the case files on 5 children (18 per cent) had already been closed. The reasons for this were as follows: In two cases further support by the Social Services Department was considered to be unnecessary. Contact with one family was lost when they moved out of the city. One child was adopted and one child died. The child who died was under a supervision order. The other four children were receiving support on a voluntary basis.

Thus, only 23 cases remained open at the time of the survey. Eighteen children (78 per cent) were living at home, 1 was still in hospital, while the other 4 were in the care of the local authority. Seventeen children (74 per cent) were receiving voluntary supervision, while 1 was under a supervision order. One child had been received into care while 4 were subjects of care orders.

SOCIAL MOBILITY

Eleven families (50 per cent) had changed their address. Five (29 per cent) had changed their family doctor. Six (26 per cent) had experienced a change of social worker dealing with the case.

CURRENT SITUATION

Improvement in the material state of the home was noted in 12 cases (55 per cent) and deterioration in one case. Improvement in the family situation was recorded for 10 cases (44 per cent) and worse for 2 cases. Co-operation was better in 11 cases (48 per cent), the same in 9 cases, and worse in 3 cases.

CHILD'S HEALTH

The social workers considered the child's general health to be better in 19 cases (83 per cent) and his general welfare to be improved in 16 cases (70 per cent). No child was reported to be in a worse state of general health or welfare.

FURTHER UNEXPLAINED INJURIES

In one third of families (7 out of 20) either the child or its siblings were suspected by the social worker of demonstrating unexplained injuries. None of these children had been removed from the home.

COMMENTS ON THE FOLLOW-UP SURVEY

The success of a follow-up survey requires the co-operation of both the subjects and those agencies that have access to information. The organization involved in launching this simple follow-up survey was considerable and a great deal of labour could have been saved, and more data obtained if it was possible to collaborate fully and continuously with all the social workers involved. The author's experience suggested that some departments jealousy guarded their information against probing by an outside investigator. It was also interesting to observe that such departments adopted a similar attitude to social workers from other areas or agencies. While the author accepts that the release of confidential information raises ethical considerations, particularly if the investigator is likely to take punitive action towards the families concerned, the obstacles placed in the path of information gathering in this survey, seemed arbitary and at times excessive. Indeed the success of a long-term follow-up study of these children is likely to be dependent on the personal contacts and individual professional affiliations of the researchers. Such considerations might save others from disappointment and wasted effort.

CHARACTERISTICS OF IDENTIFIED PERPETRATORS

Sixty parents confessed to battering their child. Forty-three of these were mothers and 17 were fathers. There were 74 cases where neither parent was identified.

PERSONALITY AND CHILD-REARING PRACTICES

Tables 27–30 compare findings for those parents who were identified as perpetrators with the total index sample and contrasts them with those parents who were not so identified. Where there was no significant difference between those parents who were identified as a perpetrator and the remainder of the index sample, the variable has been omitted from the table.

SOCIAL CHARACTERISTICS

Most of the social characteristics mentioned in Chapter 14 apply to both parents. Table 31 compares findings for those homes where either parent was identified as a perpetrator with the total sample and contrasts them with those homes where neither parent could be identified. Where there was no significant difference between homes with and without an identified perpetrator, the variable has been omitted from the table.

TABLE 27

Personality Characteristics of Identified Mother Perpetrators Compared with Total Sample and with those Unidentified as Perpetrators

Index mothers	*Total sample*		*Identified perpetrators*		*Unidentified*		*Significance*	
	No.	*Per cent*	*No.*	*Per cent*	*No.*	*Per cent*	χ^2	p*
Abnormal personality	95	(76)	38	(88)	57	(70)	4.51	< 0.05
Neurosis	60	(48)	33	(77)	27	(33)	19.6	< 0.001
Criminal record	14	(11)	2	(5)	12	(14)	Nos. too small for χ^2	
	No.	*Mean*	*No.*	*Mean*	*No.*	*Mean*	t	p
Social class	119	3.9	34	4.2	85	3.8	2.09	< 0.05
Neuroticism (EPI)	112	14.4	41	17.8	71	12.5	5.98	< 0.001
G.H.Q. (Goldberg)	83	19.2	34	31.4	49	10.8	6.14	< 0.001
H.D.H.Q. (Foulds)								
Total hostility	105	22.5	39	26.9	66	20.3	4.44	< 0.001
Acting-out hostility		4.7		5.6		4.2	2.94	< 0.01
Self-criticism		5.7		6.5		5.2	2.60	$= 0.01$
Projected hostility		2.7		3.6		2.3	2.64	< 0.01
Guilt		3.3		4.5		2.6	4.33	< 0.001

* These values are for the comparison between cases for whom a parent was identified as a perpetrator and those without such identification.

TABLE 28

Personality Characteristics of Identified Father Perpetrators Compared with Total Sample and with those Unidentified as Perpetrators

Index fathers	*Total sample*		*Identified perpetrators*		*Unidentified*		*Significance*	
	No.	*Per cent*	*No.*	*Per cent*	*No.*	*Per cent*	χ^2	p*
Abnormal personality	57	(64)	13	(87)	44	(60)	10.72	< 0.01
Criminal record	26	(29)	5	(42)	21	(2)	Nos. too small for χ^2	
	No.	*Mean*	*No.*	*Mean*	*No.*	*Mean*	t	p
Age	105	27.0	15	23.2	90	27.6	5.39	< 0.001
Wife's age	131	23.5	16	21.1	115	23.9	4.09	< 0.001
Neuroticism (EPI)	66	9.6	13	13.4	53	8.7	2.40	< 0.05
G.H.Q. (Goldberg)	54	11.0	10	25.4	44	7.7	2.80	< 0.05
H.D.H.Q. (Foulds)								
Total hostility	65	18.6	14	24.9	51	16.8	2.79	$= 0.01$
Acting out hostility		4.4		5.6		4.1	1.97	$= 0.07$
Self-criticism		3.9		5.4		3.5	2.07	$= 0.05$
Paranoid hostility		2.1		3.8		1.7	2.85	$= 0.01$
Guilt		2.2		4.1		1.7	3.05	< 0.01

*These values are for the comparison between cases for whom a parent was identified as a perpetrator and those without such identification.

TABLE 29

Recollections of Childhood of Identified Mother Perpetrators Compared with Total Sample and with those Unidentified as Perpetrators

Index mothers	*Total sample*		*Identified perpetrator*		*Unidentified*		*Significance*	
	No.	*Per cent*	*No.*	*Per cent*	*No.*	*Per cent*	χ^2	p*
Unhappy childhood	42	(34)	25	(81)	17	(52	4.72	< 0.05
Two or more neurotic symptoms	63	(51)	29	(69)	34	(42)	7.07	< 0.01
Impaired relationships with parents	43	(36)	23	(56)	20	(25)	9.82	< 0.01
Impaired relationships as a child	39	(32)	22	(51)	17	(21)	10.50	< 0.01
Impaired relationships with siblings	22	(19)	14	(37)	8	(10)	9.86	< 0.01
Physical maltreatment	31	(25)	22	(51)	9	(11)	22.32	< 0.001
Own father rejecting or harsh	36	(32)	18	(50)	18	(24)	6.13	< 0.05
Own father warm and affectionate	69	(73)	18	(54)	51	(84)	7.84	< 0.01

*These values are for the comparison between cases for whom a parent was identified as a perpetrator and those without such identification.

TABLE 30

Child-Rearing Practices of Identified Mother Perpetrators Compared with Total Sample and with those not Identified as Perpetrators

Index mothers	*Total sample*		*Identified perpetrators*		*Unidentified*		*Significance*	
	No.	*Per cent*	*No.*	*Per cent*	*No.*	*Per cent*	χ^2	p*
Frequent use of physical punishment	58	(50)	28	(67)	30	(41)	6.31	< 0.05
Praises for good behaviour	11	(10)	8	(19)	3	(4)	4.69	< 0.05
Severe potty training	12	(15)	8	(27)	4	(8)	3.92	< 0.05
Demands for instant obedience	31	(30)	17	(49)	14	(21)	7.07	< 0.01
Demands for obedience	86	(84)	32	(91)	44	(81)	5.73	< 0.05
Crying and clinging not necessarily a problem	69	(64)	33	(80)	36	(54)	6.78	< 0.01
Partner no help not necessarily a problem	47	(44)	26	(63)	21	(32)	8.64	< 0.01
Punishment for screaming	22	(29)	17	(57)	5	(11)	16.36	< 0.001
Isolation for screaming	29	(28)	6	(20)	23	(50)	5.71	< 0.05
Aggressive behaviour punished	20	(29)	12	(48)	8	(19)	5.24	< 0.05
Rigid feeding schedule	25	(22)	14	(33)	11	(15)	4.37	< 0.05
Emotional overinvolvement when child refuses food	28	(29)	19	(51)	9	(15)	13.01	< 0.001

* These values are for the comparison between cases for whom a parent was identified as a perpetrator and those without such identification.

TABLE 31

Characteristics of Homes where either Parent is an Identified Perpetrator Compared with Total Sample and with Homes Where Neither Parent has been so Identified

Information from Index mothers	*Total sample*		*Parent identified*		*No parent identified*		*Significance*	
	No.	*Per cent*	*No.*	*Per cent*	*No.*	*Per cent*	χ^2	p*
Absent father	44	(35)	27	(49)	17	(24)	7.26	< 0.01
Unsatisfactory marriage	36	(30)	26	(49)	10	(15)	15.21	< 0.001
Low opinion of partner	15	(13)	13	(21)	2	(3)	9.77	< 0.01
Disagreement over child rearing	47	(41)	32	(62)	15	(24)	15.25	< 0.001
Mother head of house	21	(15)	16	(30)	5	(8)	7.88	< 0.01
Two or more changes of address in 3 years	(Mean = 2.0 for 122 cases)		(Mean = 2.3 for 55 cases)		(Mean = 1.8 for 67 cases)		(t = 2.66)	< 0.01
Loneliness	63	(54)	15	(27)	48	(77)	13.49	< 0.001
Inadequate house-keeping allowance	44	(36)	29	(53)	15	(23)	10.41	< 0.01
Mother dissatisfied	34	(26)	26	(47)	6	(9)	20.98	< 0.001
Mother has no worries	14	(13)	2	(4)	12	(18)	4.61	< 0.05

* These values are for the comparison between cases for whom a parent was identified as a perpetrator and those without such identification.

PART IV

INTERPRETATION OF THE FINDINGS

Chapter 17

Discussion

CLINICAL CHARACTERISTICS OF THE CHILDREN

AGE

The finding that equal numbers of boys and girls were battered agrees with others (Ebbin *et al.*, 1969; Salmon, 1971) but differs from those who maintain there is a preponderance of boys (Skinner and Castle, 1969; Lukianowicz, 1971; Gil, 1970). Several authors (Schloesser, 1964; Simons *et al.*, 1966; Kempe, 1971) have commented on the younger age of battered children and assert (Skinner and Castle, 1969) that these are particularly at risk. The results from this study show that emergency admissions tend to be younger even if not battered. The results also showed that most children were under 2 years of age and a high proportion had been previously battered. These findings (and those of others) may, however, be reconciled by the observation that younger children had more serious injuries and were thus more likely to be hospitalized, thus supporting suggestions that 'any injury (other than a road traffic accident) to a child under two must be considered to be an instance of the battered baby syndrome' (Lancet, 1971). This is further exemplified by the finding that battered children were significantly younger than other emergency admissions and that the risk rapidly diminished after the age of two.

TYPES OF INJURY

The results confirm those of others who have shown that battered children have a multiplicity of injuries in various stages of healing

(Kempe *et al.*, 1962; Weston, 1968; Ebbin *et al.*, 1969). Vague accounts 'must have knocked his head against the cot', 'fell off the bed', 'bruises easily', were offered as initial explanations by parents. In no case was a bleeding disorder detected. Bruising to the head or cheek, a black eye without gross bruising of the forehead, a 'purple ear' or fading bruises of the ear and surrounding scalp were prominent features supporting those who rate the head as an important site of trauma (Skinner and Castle, 1969; Cameron, 1972).

More than one third had an intracranial haemorrhage (usually subdural) and a high proportion had no associated skull fractures. Fifteen per cent had no head bruising, but showed instead minimal finger and thumb mark bruises on the trunk and arms. These children had been shaken violently, supporting Guthkelch's suggestions (1971) that repeated acceleration/deceleration (whiplash injury), rather than direct violence, accounts for intracranial bleeding. Diagnostic confusion also arose in those children with ocular damage. Here the findings concur with others (Harcourt and Hopkins, 1971; Mushin, 1971) who have concluded that physical maltreatment must be strongly considered when intraocular haemorrhages, with or without an associated subdural effusion occurs.

Though bruises, fractures, subdural haematoma and malnutrition are being increasingly recognized as stigmata of baby battering, little emphasis has been placed on child abuse by burning. The finding that nearly 20 per cent had serious burns or scalds and that such children were significantly older than the remainder of the sample supports suggestions that many incidents of child abuse by burning pass for accidents (Stone *et al.*, 1970). The importance of skeletal surveys (repeated 2 weeks later if negative) was shown by the fact that nearly half had fractures. Cigarette burns were not common but burning of the buttocks or perineum by placing the child on a hot metal surface was a particularly striking feature – a finding also observed by Vesterdal (1972).

As expected the proportion of dead children having skull fractures, intracranial haemorrhages and abdominal injuries was greater than for the rest of the sample. Thirty-three per cent had been battered more than once. The types of injuries observed were similar to those described by others (Touloukian, 1968; Weston, 1968). The finding that 33.3 per cent had a sibling who had also been maltreated should caution against the over-optimistic belief that only one child in a family is affected (Merrill, 1962; Zalba, 1966). Considering also that most fatal cases resulted from a single act of parental violence this finding emphasizes the importance of considering a care order on other children in a family even though not yet battered.

COT DEATHS

Adelson (1961) and Emery (1972) suggest that some 'accidental' and 'cot deaths' may be victims of parental assault. Nine per cent of the index sample had a sibling who died; some of these under suspicious circumstances. Sudden infant deaths are characterized by a long delay between the child last being seen alive and the discovery of death, illegitimacy and low birth weight. Poor use of welfare service, poor living conditions, marital disharmony and poor work records characterize the parents of such children (Richards and McIntosh, 1972). In this study baby batterers shared all these adversities. Furthermore, half the sample of dead children were 'discovered' after a delay of 24 hours or longer from the injury, suggesting that some 'cot deaths' may conceivably be battered babies.

MORTALITY RATE

Mortality rates for children subjected to wilful violence varies among different series – less than 2 per cent (Skinner and Castle, 1969), 3 per cent (Gregg and Elmer, 1969), 11 per cent (Kempe 1971), 25–30 per cent (Helfer, 1968) and 55 per cent (Vesterdal, 1972). In this series the rate is 8 per cent after excluding prison cases and is most similar to the findings of Kempe (1962) and Cooper (1974). Other series in this country have also found higher rates (Hall, 1974; Mounsey, 1974); these may be due to sampling differences. If prison cases are included (which reflect a national rather than local incidence, and therefore cannot strictly be combined) the mortality rate in this series is also 16 per cent. The commonest causes of death in children aged 0–4 years are birth injuries, infections and congenital abnormalities. Apart from 'accidents', battering in Birmingham in 1971 ranked next above motor vehicle accidents as a cause of death (City of Birmingham, 1972). Other observations from this study suggest that unless medical personnel overcome their reluctance to record a diagnosis of 'battered child syndrome' (W.H.O., 1968) accurate statistics on the size of this problem will remain merely guesswork. National statistics are also hampered: in five of the cases in this series who died in Birmingham in 1971 the coroner reached an 'open verdict'. Thus none appeared in the Registrar General's figures (Registrar General, 1973) for 'homicides and injuries purposely inflicted in 1971.

NEUROLOGICAL AND INTELLECTUAL IMPAIRMENT

The findings support those of others (Helfer, 1968; Martin, 1972) who showed that battering often results in permanent neurological impairment. Fifteen per cent of the sample developed spasticity, paraplegia, blindness and other neurological sequelae that required long term rehabilitation. One child developed West's syndrome (infantile spasms, subnormality, hypsarrhythmia) following violent shaking.

The findings also show that battering leads to developmental retardation. A proportion of those tested (39 per cent) suffered head injuries that were not thought clinically to result in brain damage, yet their overall abilities were lower than for the remainder, and the personal–social and hand–eye co-ordination scales were the abilities most affected. Abnormality of social responsiveness and visuo-motor co-ordination were found in those children who had suffered only slight head injuries. Such behaviour is, therefore, probably due to CNS damage.

Ounsted (1972) has asserted that battered children are silent and gaze fixatedly ('frozen watchfulness') and suggested that this characteristic behaviour pattern results from an inability to establish basic trusting relationships with their parents. Because the capacity for showing mistrust develops slowly in early childhood (Schaffer, Greenwood and Parry, 1972) such observations in young babies may be misinterpretation. In older children immobility can be a normal response to a new experience (Schaffer, 1974) such as hospitalization. Children in this study were tested after adaptation to hospital, and only one child behaved mistrustfully throughout testing. The sample were also characterized by language retardation regardless of head injury. This has also been observed by Martin (1972).

Thirty-eight per cent of the sample were without head injury or neurological damage but their overall ability was also significantly lower than the controls. This may be due to previous head trauma or genetic endowment. Parental neglect may result in low birth weight, congenitally defective and failure to thrive babies (Crosse, 1971). That such factors may also be responsible, was supported by the finding that lower developmental quotients were obtained by children having such handicaps. Only 22 battered children (16 per cent) were without brain damage, head injury, low birth weight or failure to thrive.

Considering that most parents offer no adequate explanation of the injury and that approximately half the cases of cerebral palsy and mental deficiency attending paediatric out-patient departments have no adequate cause identified (MacKeith, 1974) the possibility that battering is responsible for a sizeable proportion needs further exploration.

PHYSICAL NEGLECT AND FAILURE TO THRIVE

Focusing on a battered child without regard to its siblings may result in disastrous consequences. This was exemplified by one mother who battered her son aged 2 years. This child was closely supervised by a health visitor and social worker who both failed to notice the development of marasmus in his sister aged 10 weeks, who had been starved and died shortly after admission to hospital (*see* Case 2, Chapter 12). Childhood marasmus as a primary nutritional disorder is, of course, not common in Britain. The possibility that it represents another form of rejection should be strongly considered for another similar case has been described recently (Talukder and Dawson, 1974).

The finding that a significant number of battered children were also physically neglected, is at variance with those who maintain that battering and neglect are mutually exclusive phenomena (Steele and Pollock, 1968). A significant proportion of the sample had been previously admitted to hospital with failure to thrive, supporting the suggestion that maltreatment of children is a spectrum ranging from murder and infanticide to physical assault, neglect and nutritional and emotional deprivation (Schloesser, 1964; Simons *et al.*, 1966; Koel, 1969; Martin, 1972). Indeed the overlap between physical neglect and failure to thrive was considerable. It was also interesting to observe that after discharge home, the children in this study failed to maintain the growth they had maintained in hospital, supporting suggestions that lack of calorie intake (Whitten, Pettit and Fischoff, 1969) or deprivation of appropriate maternal affection (Silver and Finkelstein, 1967) may impair growth and curtail intellectual development (Winick, 1969).

LOW BIRTH WEIGHT AND MOTHER'S OBSTETRIC HISTORY

Twenty-five per cent of battered children born in hospital were low birth weight babies. This figure falls to 15 per cent if the assumption be made that babies born at home were of normal weight and compares with 5–7 per cent in the population at large (Butler and Alberman, 1969; Crosse, 1971; Wadsworth, 1974). Several authors (Simons *et al.*, 1966; Gregg and Elmer, 1969; Skinner and Castle, 1969) have asserted that low birth weight babies are particularly at risk of battering and others (Klaus and Kennell, 1970; Klein and Stern, 1971) have interpreted this as failure of bonding due to separating the mother from her child during the neonatal period. The over-representation of low birth weight babies in this and other series (Simons *et al.*, 1966;

Gregg and Elmer, 1969; Skinner and Castle, 1969; Klein and Stern, 1971) may, however, be simply explained as reflecting those maternal characteristics and predispose to delivery of low birth weight babies – low social class, youthful and single status, and rejecting attitudes during pregnancy (Drillien, 1964; Crosse, 1971). All these characteristics were prevalent in this study. Newson (1973*b*) has pointed out that responsiveness to a baby is not a simple matter of biological necessity but a general characteristic shared by many people who are not mothers. Furthermore it has been demonstrated that unfavourable mother–child relationships are related to undesirable maternal attitudes long before the neonatal period (Davids and Holden, 1970) and to personality abnormality (Pohlman, 1973). Considering also that only a small proportion weighed under 2000 g at birth or required long-term separation from the mother, it is unrealistic to expect that increased or improved maternal–child contact following confinement (Klaus and Kennell, 1970; Klein and Stern, 1971) will substantially reduce the risk of subsequent battering.

No support was found for suggestions that difficulties during pregnancy, labour or post-partum (Schloesser, 1964; Steele and Pollock, 1968; Skinner and Castle, 1969) are responsible. Most had normal confinements and only a small proportion battered during the post-partum period. Indeed this study showed that many mothers had longstanding emotional and personality problems and displayed rejecting attitudes towards their children irrespective of puerperal factors.

PROVOCATION BY THE CHILD AND CONTACT WITH FAMILY PRACTITIONERS

It has been suggested that some children are particularly at risk and unwittingly invite physical abuse from their parents (Milowe and Lourie, 1964). Failure to take account of the fact that child–parent I.Q. correlations are low before the age of 3 years (Honzik, 1957) and failure to use well validated tests such as the Griffiths developmental scales (Hindley, 1965) may exaggerate the significance of clinical impressions that a child's intellectual endowment exceeds or falls short of the parents (Martin, 1972). The results showed that battered children were not hyperactive but were in some respects lethargic. Difficulty, especially crying or clinging behaviour, was encountered by the index mothers and may have precipitated battering. However, the results do not support suggestions that these children necessarily invite physical abuse since after being in hospital for some time they were not observed to be any more irritable than the controls. It is more satisfactory to regard such difficult behaviour as probably resulting from the interaction with a neurotic mother (Rutter, 1966). The results bear this out.

Kempe (1971) has asserted that in the prodromal stages mothers often and recurrently bring their infants with non-existent complaints and that family doctors are slow to identify and refer suspected cases (Skinner and Castle, 1969). The findings from this study are at variance with this, for no mother had made an unnecessary visit to her family doctor before the battering of her child. Indeed family doctors are unlikely to see more than one case in 5 years (White Franklin, 1975). More characteristic was the long delay between injury and arrival at hospital; a factor also observed in other studies (Lukianowicz, 1971; Gil, 1970).

PSYCHIATRIC CHARACTERISTICS OF THE PARENTS

AGE

The young age of mothers closely compares with the age distribution described by other authors (Gil, 1968*b*; Skinner and Castle, 1969). On average index mothers were aged 19.7 years at the birth of their first child. This compares strikingly with the national average of 23.3 years (Registrar General, 1972*a*). Even in the lowest social class the average was 22.6 years (Newson and Newson, 1963). Index mothers were thus nearly 4 years younger than the national average when they gave birth to their first infant. Considering that most battered babies were first or second born and that more than half were under 18 months old when battered it may be concluded that battering is associated with youthful parenthood. This argument is further exemplified by the infrequent occurrence of battering in older parents with large families observed in this and other series (Bennie and Sclare, 1969; Lukianowicz, 1971) and suggests that the risk of battering diminishes with parental age.

SOCIAL CLASS

The parents in this series were predominantly from the lower social classes. The association of low social class with battering parents has been commented on by several other workers (Young, 1964; Skinner and Castle, 1969). No support was found for the statement that all social classes are represented (Kempe, 1969). Of the index group 76 per cent were from social classes IV and V compared with only 32 per cent in the Birmingham population (City of Birmingham, 1972). It may be argued that such a large discrepancy is due to the youthfulness of the parents and type of admission (emergency) of the children. Nevertheless, despite allowing for these important factors it was found that the control group also contained 33 per cent of social class IV and V. This strongly suggests that battering is mainly a lower social class phenomenon. Furthermore, as the criteria for referral of cases were medical it may be reasonably assumed that if more children from high social class families had been admitted with unexplained injuries then consultant paediatricians would have referred them.

ABNORMAL PERSONALITY

Abnormality of personality was a significant finding among the parents of battered children. The less severe types of personality disturbance were more commonly found among the mothers, who in general had features of emotional immaturity and dependence. Many of these mothers had in addition little concept of appropriate child-rearing practices (*see* Chapter 15). Battering may at best be regarded as an ineffectual method of controlling their child's behaviour. Techniques of teaching child-rearing skills based realistically on their low intelligence should perhaps be explored further as a possible means of correcting such ineffectual parent care.

Among the fathers studied 33.3 per cent were psychopaths. The association of battering with psychopathy has been commented on before (Birrell and Birrell, 1968; Lukianowicz, 1971; Scott, 1973) but contrasts with Kempe's (1969) finding that psychopathy is a feature in only 2 or 3 per cent of battering parents. Though most of these fathers had not killed their children it is disconcerting to observe that they share similar personality characteristics with a group of fathers who did kill their children (Scott, 1973; Oliver, 1974).

CRIMINAL RECORDS

Twenty-nine per cent of the fathers had a criminal record. Though the follow-up period was brief, nevertheless 6.7 per cent went on to commit subsequent crimes. Furthermore though 19 per cent of the children's siblings had been previously battered only 1 per cent of the parents had been charged with cruelty or neglect, highlighting the capriciousness of the legal system towards parents who batter babies.

Criminality and recidivism particularly if associated with a psychopathic personality should caution against an optimistic outcome, and invoking a care order is essential if further battering incidents are to be prevented. No association was found with alcoholism or drug addiction, which agrees with Steele and Pollock's (1968) findings but differs from those of Young (1964) and Gil (1968*a*) who maintained that battering is precipitated by alcoholism.

NEUROSIS

It was found that mothers were neurotic by three different measures. Fifty-eight per cent were non-psychotically disturbed on Goldberg's General Health Questionnaire and 48 per cent were diagnosed as neurotic at interview – the usual symptomatology being depression, anxiety or a mixture of both. The diagnosis of neuroticism on the Eysenck Personality Inventory lends some support to the clinical finding of neurosis and the questionnaire results. Thirty-four per cent reported having an unhappy childhood. In general neurotic mothers – in contrast to psychopathic fathers – confessed to harming their children and expressed willingness to discuss their difficulties further. For this particular group of mothers the combination of symptomatic relief with a programme of social re-learning conducted by skilled therapists seems to the author to be far more beneficial than relying solely on programmes of 'mothering' and other methods (Kempe and Helfer, 1972) that tend to reinforce their dependent behaviour.

Neuroticism was also found to be an important characteristic of those mothers who confessed to battering their children. Among the fathers neuroticism was masked by the high proportion who denied battering the child. However, among the fathers who were identified as perpetrators the mean scores on both the Eysenck Personality Inventory and the General Health Questionnaire were abnormally high. The need for these parents to act out their hostility was not detected for the sample as a whole but emerged when only those who confessed to battering were singled out. This is not surprising considering that items on this scale would be particularly pointed for a battering sample – for example, 'When I'm angry I feel like smashing things'.

HOSTILITY

Foulds has shown that as a general rule the hostility of neurotics is of the introverted kind (Caine, Foulds and Hope, 1967). The results from this study, however, showed that baby batterers who were neurotic were not predominantly intropunitive, but were characterized equally by extrapunitiveness. The most clear-cut for both mothers and fathers were the bizarre forms of hostility, hitherto found only in psychiatric populations (Philip, 1969) namely projected hostility and guilt. While guilt and remorse have often been dismissed as symptoms unrelated to actual circumstances in psychiatric populations and as glib sophistication among psychopaths (Hare, 1972), there is no reason to suppose that the guilt experienced by the sample is not reality-orientated or genuine, considering recent events. Considering their impaired relationships their high level of paranoid hostility is perhaps also understandable.

The need for these parents to act out their hostility was not detected for the sample as a whole but emerged when only those who confessed to battering were singled out. This is not surprising, as items on this scale would be particularly revealing when put to a battering parent. For example, 'When I'm angry I feel like smashing things'. Self-criticism was also not detected for the sample as a whole, so that on first inspection of the results the pattern of significant types of hostility was most reminiscent of psychopaths who 'may regard themselves as hot-tempered, cynical, interestingly mad or diabolically wicked; but . . . draw the line at appearing faintly inferior or incompetent' (Philip, 1969). However, those who confessed to battering did not draw the line in their self-descriptions. This group of baby batterers may possibly, as previously suggested (Smith, Hanson and Noble, 1973, 1974), be more amenable to treatment.

Thus the results depict baby batterers as neurotic – chiefly depressed – and characterized by all kinds of hostility directed against both others and themselves. This description resembles that of the depressive psychopath (Sattes, 1972). Indeed in the backgrounds of the sample there was considerable evidence of psychiatric disturbance; childhood neurotic symptoms, childhood unhappiness, a family history of psychiatric illness, physical handicaps, head injuries and lack of school success. Despite such adversities very few baby batterers had received any formal psychiatric treatment.

PSYCHOMOTOR PERFORMANCE

The Spiral Maze

A test of risk-taking while under pressure has demonstrated that delinquents have relatively fast and careless performances, while behaviour disordered children are likely to be either fast and careless or slow and careless (Gibson, 1964). West and Farrington (1973) have pointed out that clumsiness, although significantly predictive of both juvenile delinquency and recidivism, seems to be 'of importance only because of its association with low intelligence'. It was found that index and control mothers did not differ on the 'quick and careless (to slow and accurate)' dimension but that index mothers were more slow and clumsy. The prevalence of depression in this sample probably contributed something to the slow tempo (Mayo, 1966) but the clumsiness may be regarded as a reflection of low intelligence. The relative effects of personality and intelligence on the psychomotor behaviour of baby batterers deserves more attention. However, risk-taking when under pressure does not appear, from the results of the Spiral Maze Test, to be a characteristic of battering parents.

PSYCHOSIS

The findings confirm the view that only a minority of battering parents are psychotic (Steele and Pollock, 1968). The bizarre nature of the injuries inflicted by psychotic parents suggests that they form a separate sub-group among baby batterers whose management must differ accordingly.

ABNORMAL EEGs

Because the numbers who underwent EEGs are on the small side, tentative conclusions only may be drawn from this aspect of the study. Nevertheless, the prevalence of abnormal EEG findings strongly suggests that some baby batterers at least are much more closely related to other groups committing acts of violence than they are to the general population. This is borne out also by the results of psychological testing, particularly of the group with abnormal EEGs, which also showed a consistent variation from the normal population. It would, therefore, seem clear that baby batterers are not a homogenous group about whom it is safe to generalize. Whereas in some instances battering may be a response to unusual and excessive stress situations – though this needs further investigation – the presence of a definitely abnormal EEG in almost 25 per cent of cases points to what may well be a separate sub-group to which special attention should be paid. This is further borne out by a demonstrable relationship between personality diagnosis and abnormal EEGs. Indeed 5 female batterers and 1 male batterer all with abnormal EEGs could undoubtedly be classed not only as having a personality disorder, but as aggressive psychopaths (Walton and Presly, 1973). The male subject also had a criminal record. The two other female patients exhibited a personality disorder though this was not primarily of an aggressive type.

VIOLENCE BREEDS VIOLENCE?

Steele and Pollock (1968) have suggested that baby batterers were deprived both of basic mothering and of the deep sense of being cared for from the beginning of their lives. Some of the findings from this study are at variance with this suggestion. Significant proportions of index mothers said they were physically maltreated in childhood and that their parents were unreasonable, rejecting and harsh. High proportions of index fathers also experienced punitiveness from their own parents, and significant proportions said their parents were unreasonable in their disciplinary methods, supporting those authors (Gibbens and Walker, 1956; Tuteur and Glotzer, 1966; Steele and Pollock, 1968; Fontana, 1968) who suggested that such child-rearing practices reflected childhood experiences. On the other hand the sample did not report lack of affection to any greater extent than others of low social class. Considering the parents were willing to report unreasonable discipline, there is no reason to assume that lack of affection was not reliably reported. Such inconsistencies may be realistic illustrations of the backgrounds of baby batterers.

SOCIAL CHARACTERISTICS

LACK OF FAMILY COHESIVENESS

The findings from this study also suggest that lack of family cohesiveness is an important factor underlying baby battering. In over 33.3 per cent of cases the biological father was absent from the home and in 50 per cent the mothers were living with some other man. These findings closely agree with those of several other authors (Simons *et al.*, 1966; Gil, 1970; Fontana, 1971) and are at variance with those who maintain that battering parents have stable personal relationships (Steele and Pollock, 1968).

Fifty per cent of the mothers in the index sample had married before the age of 20 years and 75 per cent had conceived pre-maritally. Among the population at large such a combination is particularly likely to be associated with marital breakdown (Rowntree, 1964; Goode, 1966). Though fewer index than control parents directly admitted marriage problems a significant proportion reported disharmony in child-rearing and dissatisfaction with the partner's handling of the child. These characteristics may be taken as indices of disagreement between husband and wife over their respective roles; such indices are also predictors of divorce (Goode, 1966). Short acquaintance before marriage is another predictor of divorce found in the sample. Fifty per cent of the mothers were neurotic and 66.6 per cent of the fathers had a personality disorder. Neurotic and personality disorders are factors also associated with marital breakdown (Burgess and Wallin, 1953; Kreitman *et al.*, 1970). In contrast in early marriages the kinship support has been shown to be an important contributory force in stabilizing the marriage (de Lissovoy, 1973). However, the parents in this study had little contact with their own parents and other relatives. Considering, therefore, that a significant proportion suffered all these marital adversities and that 33.3 per cent of battered babies were already living with one natural parent only, it may be predicted that a substantial number will eventually grow up in broken homes.

Broken homes, unhappy homes and one-parent families are associated with delinquency (Glueck and Glueck, 1962; Gibson, 1969), deviant behaviour (Rutter, 1971) and social and education deprivation (Crellin *et al.*, 1971) respectively. The author's sample has a very large share of such predictors of maldevelopment in the child. Fatal battering has been shown to occur where young, unstable, deserted and unhappy women associate with young, psychopathic and criminal men (Scott, 1973). Such parents were over-represented in this study suggesting that battered children are at risk not only of social maldevelopment but also of fatal injury.

PRE-MARITAL CONCEPTION AND ILLEGITIMACY

A high proportion of index mothers conceived pre-maritally and more than 33.3 per cent of battered children were illegitimate. This finding is in close agreement with that of other investigations both in the United States (Merrill, 1962; Simons *et al.*, 1966; Bennie and Sclare, 1969) and in the United Kingdom (Gibbens and Walker, 1956; Lukianowicz, 1971). The findings are also particularly striking in the light of those studies (Weir, 1970; Crellin *et al.*, 1971) which showed that pre-marital pregnancy and illegitimacy are not simply (or directly) related to social class. This was also borne out by the observation that equating index and control sample for class did not reduce the contrast between them. Among the population at large the highest proportion of pre-maritally conceived and illegitimate births is found between 15 and 19 years of age and then decreases with maternal age (Crellin *et al.*, 1971; Registrar General, 1973, Part 2. The mothers in this study, however, differed in this respect; the highest proportion of such births occurring in those between 25 and 34 years. Furthermore, in all age groups studied the mothers have strikingly more pre-marital pregnancies and illegitimate births than the general population (Registrar General, 1973, Part 2). The highest proportion of all were aged between 20 and 24 years. The rates of occurrence of pre-marital pregnancy and illegitimacy were two and three times respectively higher than the general population rates. The findings strongly suggest, therefore, that pre-marital conception and illegitimacy are important precursors of baby battering. It is disconcerting to observe that illegitimacy was present in 60 per cent of Weston's fatal battered baby cases (Weston, 1968) and that the inconvenience of an unwanted illegitimate child was the most common motive responsible for child murder (Resnick, 1969).

UNWANTED CONCEPTION

Though displeasure at pregnancy was reported by 20 per cent of index mothers, they were not atypical of their social class in this respect. A smaller but nevertheless significant proportion described their partners as currently rejecting the child and this was not class linked. Several authors (Nurse, 1966; Elmer, 1967; Lukianowicz, 1971; Vesterdal, 1972) have postulated an association between unwanted conception and baby battering but there have been no previous controlled investigations of this suggestion. Attempts to do so may, therefore, appear to document the obvious. Nevertheless, research into feelings of unwantedness is fraught with difficulties (Pohlman, 1973). It may be argued that parents who have confessed to battering a child will rationalize their behaviour by recalling that conception was unwanted. In the index sample, those parents who confessed to battering reported as much displeasure at the pregnancy as those parents who denied it.

A degree of ambivalence about pregnancy is common in the population at large (Colman and Colman 1971) and was also observed in the control sample. Harsh childhood experiences have been assumed to be responsible for lack of maternal feelings among baby batterers (Steele and Pollock, 1968). The findings suggest, that while failure to adjust to the parental role also occurs among the population at large (Jenkins, 1954) it happens more frequently among baby batterers and can be more simply understood in the context of pre-marital conception, illegitimacy and marital disharmony, rather than by linking it directly to harsh childhood experiences.

CONTRACEPTION AND ABORTION – A METHOD FOR REDUCING BABY BATTERING?

A high proportion of out-of-wedlock pregnancies are unwanted (Osborn 1963; Pohlman, 1973; Horobin, 1973). Kempe and Helfer (1972) have asserted that the most effective way to prevent battering of children is to prevent unwanted births. Several authors (Gil, 1970; Caffey, 1972; Calef, 1972) have suggested that pre-natal training for motherhood, ready availability of contraceptives, abortion on demand and encouragement of sterilization after the birth of the third child, can be important factors in the prevention of child abuse. However, there have been no controlled studies demonstrating that early and complete sex education, including contraceptive information, has led to any decline in unwanted conceptions (Hartley, 1971). Indeed, in Sweden the illegitimacy rates actually increased following the introduction of such a programme. The evidence also suggests that knowledge about the availability of contraceptives also offers no ready solution (Hartley, 1971), for in fact, the recent increases in illegitimacy rates in England, United States and Jamaica have occurred despite such increasing knowledge and availability.

The proportion of illegitimate births rose sharply over the 1950s and 1960s (Weiss, 1970) and the younger the mother's age group the greater the rise in proportion (Russell, 1970). Child abuse as observed in this study, is associated with both illegitimacy and prematurity of parenthood and these findings cannot be accounted for by social class. Although it cannot be proved that child abuse has increased over the last two decades, its clear association with both illegitimacy and teenage parenthood suggests that a real increase in child abuse may have occurred. The simplest explanation of the rise in illegitimacy rates, especially among teenagers, is that society's changing attitude has encouraged extra-marital sexual activity. An effective reversal, therefore, of those attitudes to sex and family life which are responsible for increasing rates of illegitimacy might conceivably lead to a decline in the numbers of battered babies.

Although society may facilitate or impede the availability of abortion of unwanted conceptions the evidence suggests (Davis, 1973; Horobin, 1973) that abortion will only produce a reduction in unwanted births if the motivation for limiting family size already exists.

The same argument holds for sterilization (Pohlman, 1973). The finding that a significant proportion of battering parents expressed a negative attitude towards contraception and that only 12 per cent of mothers might have even considered an abortion suggests that the preventative methods outlined by Gil (1970) and Caffey (1972), admirable though some of them may be, will have very little impact in preventing baby battering. Indeed, considering that quite as many of the index as of the control parents were in fact using some form of contraceptive, it is perhaps somewhat unrealistic to expect battering parents to become enthusiastic about birth control. The author's pessimistic view that such parents are ineffective in and distrustful of birth control is shared by Oliver and Taylor (1971) and is also supported by the finding that the battering sample, unlike the controls, were well on the way to perpetuating the large size of their family of origin.

ORDINAL POSITION OF BATTERED CHILDREN

Among the sample 33.3 per cent of the battered babies were first born and only children and 66.6 per cent of the battered babies were second and subsequent born children. Lukianowicz (1971) and others (Bennie and Sclare, 1969; Gil 1970) have suggested that it is usually the only or youngest child in a family who is battered. The battering sample bears out this trend. This, however, may be reconciled with the general tendency for infants to be hospitalized more frequently than older children (Cross, 1973). Indeed, when birth order is properly related to family size, the suggestion that a child's particular ordinal position carries more risk of battering does not hold. Furthermore the finding that 19 per cent of the child's siblings had also been battered are at variance with Zalba's (1966) assertion and Merrill's (1962) result that only one particular child in a family is abused.

ACCOMMODATION

Several American authors (Young, 1964; Sattin and Miller, 1971; Cherry and Kuby, 1971) have regarded sub-standard living accommodation as a particularly important stress that contributes to baby battering. Cherry and Kuby (1971) vividly describe their apartments 'as drab, dark and frequently foul-smelling', and most of Young's (1964) families were living in cold vermin infested and overcrowded rooms that lacked modern conveniences. In the United Kingdom several authors (Gibbens and Walker, 1956; Skinner and Castle, 1969; Scott, 1973) have also mentioned that accommodation problems are important stress factors operating within these families. In this study dilapidation was not a significant feature. Dirty and untidy homes and cramped sleeping accommodation were more common than in the control group, but when adjustments were made for social class the contrast was no longer significant. Lack of one or more essential amenities and possession of a child's own room were, however, still significant findings when the comparison was class-comparable. Nevertheless, the families in this study are not the most handicapped even in this respect, for in a sample of 'inadequate' families (Phillips, Wilson and Herbert, 1972) who had not battered their children 96 per cent lacked one or more basic amenities; a considerably higher proportion than in the author's sample. The results should therefore caution against the optimistic belief (Gil, 1970) that re-housing will reduce the prevalence of baby battering, since, on the whole, families in this study were no worse off than others of low social class. This argument is also supported by the observation (Gibbens and Walker, 1956; Skinner and Castle, 1969) that re-housing although providing temporary relief from external pressures may actually precipitate battering incidents. The findings suggest, therefore, that personality disorders frequently observed among such parents in this and other studies (Scott, 1973) are more important than environmental factors in contributing to child abuse.

RELIGION

The findings support those of others who have suggested that baby battering is not related to any particular religious affiliation (Boardman, 1962; Lukianowicz, 1971). No support, however, was found for Steele's (1968) statement that proportionately more baby batterers belong to strong, rigid, authoritatian and 'fundamentalist' types of religions. Indeed most of the parents were of nominal religion only. However, although both they and a similar proportion of control parents lacked a personal faith, it was nevertheless interesting to observe that proportionately fewer battering parents retained the personal faith of their parents. In the context of hypotheses about a battering parent's own deprived childhood experiences, lack of a persisting religious influence may be a factor worthy of further exploration.

ETHNIC FACTORS

Twenty per cent of the battered children were non-White, compared with 15 per cent non-White children aged 5 years and under in the Birmingham population at large (City of Birmingham, 1972). Owing to communication difficulties the sample did not include all Asian battered babies and the numbers on this are probably an underestimate. Nevertheless, Schloesser (1964) and Kempe (1969) have asserted that baby battering is not related to ethnic or cultural factors, in contrast to several other American studies (Simons *et al.*, 1966; Ebbin *et al.*, 1969) which have demonstrated that proportionately more battered children are coloured. However, information on the ethnic background of battered children in the United Kingdom has been limited and for this reason a comparison with the United States may not be valid. Skinner and Castle (1969) observed that 6.5 per cent of their sample were West Indian and Asian, while Scott (1973) in a study of fatal battered baby cases observed that 10 per cent of the fathers were coloured and a high proportion were Irish, but neither author reported control figures. The slight over-representation of non-White battered children in this study may reflect a higher morbidity of non-White groups. It may also be a reflection of the particular characteristics of the ethnic group concerned (Pollak, 1972). The author found no support for Gil's (1970) suggestion that the over-representation of non-White children indicates discriminating attitudes and practices on the part of the referring agency. No support either was found for suggestions that Asians and West Indians are younger, have more children and live in poorer conditions than parents of White battered babies.

Battering among West Indians may be a reflection of the higher incidence of broken homes (absence of natural father) and excessive use of physical punishment. Although few Asians had broken homes they more frequently lacked the support of contact with their parents. Thus lack of support was common to both Asian and West Indian groups.

Ebbin *et al.*, (1969) have suggested that the type of injury inflicted is not related to ethnic factors. The findings from this study concur with this statement. Of the battering group 4 mothers were psychotic, 2 being paranoid schizophrenics. Both were West Indians who inflicted bizarre injuries. Although the preference for male children in Moslem cultures is strong (Soddy, 1964) the author did not find more Moslem girls than boys in the sample.

FINANCIAL FACTORS

Financial problems have been regarded as an important precipitant of baby battering (Birrell and Birrell, 1968; Gil, 1970). However, when compared with samples of similar age and social class the income and expenditure on food of the battering group was not low. Unemployment was a characteristic of index fathers, but was no less frequent in the controls and does not therefore have the significance attributed to it by others (Skinner and Castle, 1969). It is thus erroneous to conclude that the provision of economic security to battering families by such mechanisms as 'mother's wages', 'children's allowances', 'negative income tax' (Gil, 1970) and of 'homemaker services' (Kempe and Helfer, 1972) will markedly reduce the prevalence of baby battering. In this and other related fields (Wedge and Prosser, 1973), considerable emphasis has been placed upon the relief of material hardships to the exclusion of less easily eradicated handicaps. The Children and Young Persons Act (1963) makes provision for 'giving assistance in kind or in exceptional circumstances in cash' to deserving families. However, even when aid is granted from public assistance agencies it does not prevent baby battering, for in Gil's series (Gil, 1970) nearly 66.6 per cent of the parents had received financial assistance during or prior to the year of the battering incident. It is the author's contention, therefore, that constitutional personality differences are more fundamental than financial factors in the causation of baby battering.

SOCIAL ISOLATION

Though loneliness was reported by many index mothers it was also reported by many controls, especially in the low social classes. More than 50 per cent of the index mothers lacked social contacts with neighbours and friends. Among the population at large this is also a feature that characterizes working class families, who, in contrast to middle class families, compensate for this deficiency by maintaining contact with their parents and other relatives (Willmott and Young, 1960). However, a significant proportion of the sample did not compensate in this respect and were devoid of all forms of social contact. Although social isolation may be dependent upon geographical mobility (Schaffer and Schaffer, 1968), a more significant association occurred in the sample between lack of social contact with parents and an unhappy childhood, and this may also be a reflection of the poor relationship such mothers had with their own parents. Unlike other socially-isolated populations (Schaffer and Schaffer, 1968), the battering parents did not avail themselves of social support at crisis times even though 66.6 per cent had previous contact with social agencies. Social isolation and a reluctance to avail themselves of social support had also been observed in other battered baby studies (Young, 1964; Nurse, 1966; Davoren, 1968). Nurse (1966) has asserted that because battering parents do not turn to society for help society must seek out and help battering parents. This would seem to be true, but it is unrealistic to expect such parents to take the initiative and avail themselves of 24-hour life-line services (Kempe and Helfer, 1972) operating on the lines of the Samaritans (Stengel, 1964).

Working class populations have fewer social activities (Gorer, 1955; Willmott and Young, 1960; Newson and Newson, 1963). The proportion of mothers in this study who were devoid of social activity is even higher than expected for their social class and this concurs with the finding of those authors (Nurse, 1966; Davoren, 1968) who have maintained that community contacts of battering parents are minimal. However, the contrast between mothers and their spouses in this respect is striking, for only 3 fathers did not manage to occupy their leisure time. Considering that nearly 50 per cent of mothers lacked baby-sitting arrangements and that this result was not affected by controlling for class, it could be argued that this was the prime reason for their failure to occupy themselves socially in the community. It is more probable, however, that this failure to participate in recreational activities is a reflection of the incompatability between parents themselves. This in itself may be partially explained by the high frequency of psychopathy in the fathers and neuroticism and subnormality in the mothers. In the course of this research it was found that a semantic differential technique (Osgood, Suci and Tannenbaum, 1957) was a useful means of communicating with battering parents. Psychotherapy which concentrates on the parents' perception of themselves in relation to others, taking into account their low intelligence, should be explored further as a method of relieving the mother's loneliness and possibly preventing baby battering.

The results also showed that when only those cases with a perpetrator were considered, all the social characteristics described above, with the exception of loneliness, applied to at least the same proportion. Marital disharmony emerged as particularly characteristic of the known perpetrators and this finding merits further exploration.

CHILD-REARING PRACTICES

Baby batterers have been regarded as exhibiting a specific pattern of child-rearing, characterized by demands for premature high performance and a disregard for the child's limited abilities (Steele and Pollock, 1968; Bain, 1963; Korsch *et al.*, 1965; Gregg, 1968). Such parents, being deprived of mothering in childhood (Morris and Gould, 1963; Goldston, 1965) and undergoing harsh childhood experiences (Steele and Pollock, 1968) consider punishment a proper disciplinary measure (Wasserman, 1967; Young, 1964) and look to the child for satisfaction of their own emotional needs (Morris and Gould, 1963); such characteristics being independent of age and social class (Steele and Pollock, 1968). By way of contrast punitiveness and non-permissiveness are more common among working than middle class parents (Sears *et al.*, 1957; Newson and Newson, 1968; Phillips, Wilson and Herbert, 1972) and intolerance in child-rearing is prevalent among very young parents (de Lissovoy, 1973).

Having controlled for age, the results showed that battering parents did not practice early toilet training, restrictiveness over property, rigid feeding schedules or strictness with regard to aggressive behaviour. After making further allowances for their predominantly low social class the results showed that severity of toilet training, intolerance of screaming and punishment of aggression had also – as characteristics peculiar to battering parents – to be dismissed.

However, battering parents were found to use physical punishment far more than was to be expected for their age and class. This suggests that they are 'undercontrolled' rather than 'overcontrolled' aggressors (Megargee, 1966). Mothers were also characterized by being punitive on other indices; in their tendency to use love-withdrawal as a sanction against misbehaviour, in their use of material rewards (pacifiers) and in their demands for obedience. At the same time they were relatively careless over the whereabouts or well-being of their child. Similar inconsistent attitudes are repeatedly found in the histories of other types of deviants (McCord, McCord and Zola, 1959; Robins 1966; West and Farrington, 1973). It is also instructive to note – considering the likelihood that baby batterers are transmitting their childhood experiences to their own children – that Farrington and West (1971) found undervigilance to be an even more important predictor of violent delinquency than of delinquency in general. Inconsistency towards the child on the part of the mother has not previously received comment in battered baby studies, but should perhaps be considered as providing a clue to their failure in child management.

Malone (1966) has observed that children living in dangerous environments have certain 'areas of hypertrophied ego functioning' – precocious ability. The child makes decisions for the parents and takes care of them and younger siblings. This precocious behaviour is reinforced by parental demands. Others (Davoren, 1968; Martin, 1972) have noted that some battered children are bright, precocious and capable of responding in a mature fashion to their parents' needs. The results from this study, however, showed that battered children were no more likely to be socially precocious in relation to their general development level than were the control children.

Morris and Gould (1963) have remarked that the 'concept of role reversal is necessary' for an understanding of the parents' behaviour. These authors suggest that such parents are provoked into battering because they feel unloved, unhappy and anxious when the child cries or misbehaves. To date there has been only one replicable investigation of this hypothesis, by Melnick and Hurley (1969), which suggested that mothers who batter babies have severely frustrated dependency needs and an inability to empathize with their children. This conclusion was, however, based upon only 10 cases of suspected child abuse, 8 of whom were Negro. This study has explored Morris' and Gould's concept by a semantic differential technique constructed specifically to enable parents to articulate their reactions to difficult behaviour in the child. The results showed that although their children exhibited dependent behaviour which upset the mothers more frequently, the control mothers felt equally unhappy on the occasions when such behaviour occurred. Frequency of occurrence of dependent behaviour in the child was significant, however, and was associated with maternal neuroticism in the index sample.

The differences between index mothers and index fathers and between types of problems for both index and control mothers showed that the Semantic Differential test was capable of discriminating between groups of subjects and groups of problems. However, the differences the test was designed to explore were based on suggestions in the literature relating to battered children; these did not emerge. Furthermore index and control parents did not differ in their patterns of reactions to problems with the child.

It was most interesting and important to discover that index mothers (in common with the control mothers) reacted more negatively to difficulties with their marriage than to difficulties with the child. This finding is reminiscent of the discussion in a previous section of this book (*see* Social Isolation, pp. 209–210) that marital problems and an inability to get on with adults were more significant than most material and economic problems. Inter-personal difficulties re-emerged when problems with the spouse were discussed in the context of child-rearing. It may be argued, considering that baby batterers assumed their parental roles prematurely, that their hostility is based not on rejection of the child as such, but rather on a rejection of their unsatisfactory social, marital and parental roles. The finding that index mothers had problems with their partners, especially those concerned with their lack of support in child-rearing, more frequently than the controls, deserves further study. They – as indeed did the controls – reacted more negatively to spouse than to child problems. The results suggest, therefore, that it would be more fruitful to concentrate on a battering parent's general dissatisfaction, neuroticism and hostility towards other adults, than on such phenomena as a need to be nurtured by the child.

The results also showed that battering parents were deficient in realistic attitudes towards the child – for example, in the sentiment that a child is enjoyable on the whole but that relief is welcome at times. Instead they tended to say that either they did not enjoy the child, or (more commonly), that the child meant everything to them. They were also deficient in the normal practice of allowing the child to cry for a while unless something was obviously wrong. They were instead either unresponsive or excessively responsive to crying. As well as having problems with the child's clinging behaviour, battering mothers became emotionally overinvolved when their child refused food. Despite their emotional overinvolvement there was a lack of demonstrativeness in the sample. On the whole perpetrators did not differ from the total battered baby sample of parents in their child-rearing practices. However, some already significant findings were intensified and some differences which were insignificant for the group as a whole emerged as significant when identified perpetrators were selected for comparison. These were for the latter group, severe potty training and rigid feeding schedules. (*see* Chapter 16).

Considering all the variables outlined in this chapter, battering by mothers was most clearly linked with punitiveness, carelessness in supervision, emotional overinvolvement, neuroticism, abnormal personality, hostility, marital unhappiness and adverse childhood experiences. For father's punitiveness, abnormal personality, hostility and neuroticism were important characteristics.

MANAGEMENT ASPECTS

Recent comments (New Society, 1973) have suggested that social workers have been 'too soft' and have often misjudged situations because of their enthusiasm for keeping the child and family together. Medical personnel are, however, also reluctant to notify authority particularly if they consider that this might result in parents being prosecuted. This reluctance may, of course, partly be due to the fact that medical and social welfare considerations on the one hand, and legal rights and safeguards on the other, are often hard to reconcile. However, by reserving to themselves this discretion of whether to pass on relevant information the doctor or social worker concerned may deprive the child of his legal rights of protection.

The results showed that there was a failure to ensure protection of the child. It was disconcerting to observe that the majority of cases were not brought to the attention of the juvenile court, reliance instead being placed on voluntary supervision. In view of the high mortality and morbidity reported in this and other series (Helfer, 1968; Hall, 1975; White Franklin, 1975) and the high frequency of re-battering that occurs, it is alarming to observe that no arrangements for supervision took place in 21 instances. It is the author's opinion that local authorities are failing in their statutory role of protecting the child by being reluctant to institute care proceedings.

The quality and quantity of supervision available varies in different areas, and may, of course, influence a local authority's plan of management. Nevertheless, supervision whether it be voluntary or by court order does not overcome the inherent difficulty in managing these cases – namely, that no supervisor can be with the child or his family for more than a fraction of the time. Social workers in their desire to help parents and keep families together may embark upon a programme of casework. Considerable emphasis has been placed upon intensive casework with families since the passing of the Children and Young Persons Act, 1963. The success of this has never been systematically evaluated. Furthermore management at present is hampered, in the author's opinion, by the local authorities' practice of imposing a dual role on the social worker. By appearing as the person who had made an application to deprive the parents of their parental rights, the social worker's task of establishing and pursuing a therapeutic relationship is made even more difficult. In the light of the findings from this study it is already apparent that casework will not succeed in many instances and that trusting the parents unduly may have damaging consequences to the child.

Management of the problem has in the past too often been plagued by a tendency to rely on the case conference on the assumption that discussion alone is in the child's best interests. It has been the author's experience, however, that this method is often extremely inefficient. I would propose instead that a regional team, hospital based, consisting of a paediatrician, psychiatrist, social worker and psychologist should be established to tackle the overall problem.

An alternative but somewhat complementary scheme has been proposed by Bevan (1975) who suggests that a new office of 'Children's

Guardian' should be created. The guardian would be a social worker with some legal training whose primary duty would be the protection of children's rights. Either of these appointments would perhaps improve the poor liaison that presently exists between the various agencies which concurrently and sequentially are involved in managing a case. It would also circumvent the unilateral action that often occurs through these agencies and go some way towards overcoming the present practice of returning the children home where re-battering takes place.

Other remedies rest with the courts. The case in the juvenile court is a civil and not a criminal one. It is not the court's duty to establish whether a particular individual has inflicted the injuries. It is only necessary to prove that a state of neglect or injury exists and that the parents are not preventing this. At present juvenile court magistrates have no powers to either request a psychiatric report or to recommend where appropriate that parents attend a treatment centre. It is the author's belief that improvements in child care would come about if magistrates were granted these powers.

In deciding upon an appropriate sentence, the court can follow the Criminal Justice Act, 1972 (and its amendments) which gives it wide powers – particularly if the accused has not previously been in prison. In order to decide whether other measures are more appropriate in dealing with the offender – for example, probation with a condition of treatment – the court is empowered to obtain psychiatric and social reports. This procedure allows an opportunity for reaching a sentence determined in the best interests of all concerned.

The methods used by the courts in sentencing baby batterers in this study varied. Probation with a condition of psychiatric treatment was the most frequent method used in the case of the mothers, while for fathers, imprisonment was the more likely outcome. This difference in sentencing may be due to the higher incidence of previous criminality among the fathers. It could be argued that as adult courts already have these wide powers there is no need to provide juvenile court magistrates with similar ones. However, the hesitation of doctors and social workers to facilitate criminal investigation procedures, the legal rights of the parent to remain silent and to have certain prejudicial evidence excluded and the high burden of proof on the part of the prosecution to prove their case, may all go some way towards explaining why the majority of these parents did not appear in the adult courts. Observations during this study revealed that a surprising lack of liaison occurs between the juvenile and adult courts. Furthermore, a mistaken belief is often apparent that it would be improper to mention any other proceedings in connection with the same set of facts. It is the author's belief that if the juvenile court also had the power to request psychiatric reports on the parents it would overcome some of these difficulties.

Chapter 18

Concluding Comments

In terms of morbidity and mortality the battered child is a problem of major concern to society. Oliver and Cox (1973) showed that the tendency to perpetuate child abuse in successive generations is not diminished by supplying extensive medical and social help to battering parents. Furthermore, 60 per cent of children who are returned home are re-battered (Skinner and Castle, 1969). While every effort must be made to rehabilitate battering parents this should not be at the expense of the safety of the child. The findings from this study also suggest that strong consideration should be given to permanent removal from parental care in those cases where after an overall psychiatric assessment the likelihood of parents responding to treatment is thought to be remote.

The results showed that when a variety of social and economic factors are carefully examined, baby batterers are observed to be far less handicapped than previous studies have indicated. Furthermore, when placed alongside the high incidence of personality disorders, anomalies of marital status and youthfulness of the parents, socio-economic support to such families will only be meaningful if included in a programme of adaptation to such handicaps.

The findings also suggest that it may be wrong, even dangerous so far as the children are concerned, to rely too heavily on seemingly facile explanations of why parents batter their children. There is an over-ready tendency to assume that battering parents have experienced inadequate mothering in their own childhood and are, therefore, recreating in their own child-rearing practices the same maltreatment they themselves experienced as children (Steele and Pollock, 1968). This should be avoided. Retrospective assumptions of this kind are attractive in that they are difficult to disprove. They are also, however, equally difficult to prove. To assume that all such parents or even the great majority can be adequately treated by 'a transfusion of mothering', as has been suggested (Court and Kerr, 1971; Kempe and Helfer, 1972), may not be altogether justified and in the light of the findings may even be dangerous to the children concerned.

The similarities between baby battering and other forms of deviant behaviour are striking. Like delinquency and crime in general, baby battering occurs alongside a constellation of other social inadequacies or failure of adaptation rather than in isolation. Such consideration might save some disappointment and wasted effort. Innumerable studies of deviant behaviour have been remarkably unrewarding in establishing either causes or treatment. Battering parents must first be properly classified and the natural history of the condition closely observed before we can be confident about treatment measures other than emergency action. Indeed, no study has convincingly shown that any treatment of battering parents is effective.

Child abuse has elicited spasmodic public concern for nearly a century, and yet no child protection service has so far developed that adequately meets the scope of the problem. Indeed it almost seems as if the medical profession may have abdicated its responsibility to local authorities and voluntary organizations, whose roles in some respects are complementary but in others may not always be harmonious. Both agencies rely heavily upon inexperienced and possibly inadequately-trained social workers who are as yet ill-equipped to deal with these difficult cases. The past year has again witnessed a depressing number of children who have been battered to death following decisions by social workers to return the child home. The findings from this study indicate that such authority should be curtailed. Indeed, there seems to be a strong case for setting up specialized hospital teams to carry out full assessments, giving priority to the safety and healthy development of the child. Such a team would be guided by the ethical consideration that governs all doctors – the child is at risk, the child is the patient and all other considerations are secondary.

Our knowledge is insufficient to predict which individual child will be battered. Nevertheless, the results from this and other studies broadly delineate those groups in the community which are most likely to encompass child abuse. Furthermore, the findings support Polansky's view (1968) that this is 'an area in which social, medical and legal action must be authoritative, intrusive and insistent'. As with crime and delinquency, treatment is only likely to be a supporting exercise. Prevention may rely upon adequately designed, intensive education in children's needs and development, during and following the antenatal stage. The high proportion of abnormalities at birth in this and other battered baby samples stresses the need to persuade these mothers to avail themselves of medical care. Without expert approaches to both these problems it is apparent that nearly all abused children are at risk of physical, educational and social maldevelopment or death.

In spite of some progress in strengthening the social and legal status of maltreated children the problem of child abuse continues. The battered child syndrome presents many difficult problems of recognition and management. Because the outcome of a particular case depends so much upon co-ordination and communication between the multiple professional groups that may be involved with these children, it is apparent that baby battering is a problem now ripe for review.

APPENDICES

Appendix A

METHOD AND SCOPE OF THE STUDY

PROCEDURE

In November 1970, a letter was circulated to paediatricians, accident surgeons, casualty officers and other interested agencies in the Birmingham region by Dr. Christie Gordon, Senior Administrative Officer of the West Midlands Regional Health Authority. The letter outlined the important need for research into the battered baby phenomenon and the author's particular interest in this field. Shortly after this letter was circulated the author spent several weeks outlining the objectives of the study to these professional groups. The first case was referred in January 1971.

The first consideration for a child's inclusion in the study was that in the opinion of a medically qualified person the injuries in question were inadequately explained by the parents. Parents who confessed to causing their child's injuries were also included. Doctors were asked not to take into account the appearance or background of the family as these were some of the items that were to be explored in the study. Parents were informed by the paediatrician, that the author would like to interview them as he was conducting a survey of parents of children with injuries.

A telephone appointment was made with the parents immediately after the child's admission to hospital. The author explained to the parents that he was conducting a confidential study concerned with children with similar injuries to their child and the types of problems their parents may have because of this. It was pointed out that co-operation in the study would have no particular advantage or disadvantage to them personally but that the findings might be of benefit to other children. Following their agreement each parent was then separately interviewed. A similar procedure was adopted with the controls.

DATA COLLECTION

The author spent approximately 1 hour with each parent in turn and completed the 'Circumstances of Injury/Illness' schedule first and then the 'Psychiatric Interview' schedule. At the completion of these interviews, Goldberg's General Health Questionnaire was administered. Index parents were then allocated to a group:

Group 1. Child undoubtedly battered. Parent has confessed or court has convicted parent.
Group 2. High degree of suspicion. Injury is incompatible with explanation offered.
Group 3. Some suspicion. Explanation is not quite plausible.
Group 4. Injury undoubtedly accidental.

Groups 1 and 2 only were then asked to participate in further research. Groups 3 and 4 were excluded from further interviews.

Appointments were then made for the parents to see the team's psychologist and social worker. Index parents only were also asked whether they would undergo an electroencephalogram.

Details of injuries, skeletal surveys, haematological investigations and other items contained in the 'Additional Data' schedule were then completed. The only items of information passed to the other team members were, the child's name, age, date of admission, hospital ward and the salient injuries/illnesses of the child. Parents' names and addresses were also disclosed.

The psychologist met the parents immediately or very soon afterwards and conducted the following tests separately with each parent.

(*1*) A short form of the Wechsler Adult Intelligence Scale (WAIS)
(*2*) Vineland Social Maturity Scale.
(*3*) Difficult Times Test and Semantic Differential.
(*4*) Eysenck Personality Inventory.
(*5*) Foulds Hostility and Direction of Hostility Questionnaire.
(*6*) Gibson's Spiral Maze.

Children were seen by the psychologist soon after admission and assessed on the Griffith's Mental Developmental Scales as soon as the immediate effects of their injuries had passed. Children permanently damaged were not tested.

The social worker visited the parents at home and completed a separate interview schedule with each parent. Some fathers and a few mothers were interviewed at hospital rather than not at all. Stringent precautions were taken to preserve the privacy of case records, so that no individual could be harmed by leakage of information gathered throughout the course of the study.

A large schedule of information was recorded necessitating three to four interviews with a parent, each an hour or so in duration. The response was variable but with persistence, information was obtained from most of the parents. The ambience of the hospital undoubtedly played a major part in securing the parents' co-operation. The study was also planned to counter unwillingness in several ways; the method in which the study was introduced to the parents, stressing that the study was confidential, and that the parents were contributing to research and conducting the interviews before the intervention of other agencies. Parents were also motivated by placing personal questions either at the end of an interview or interspersing them with material which was more relevant to their child's hospitalization – for example difficulties with the child followed from a general discussion of the child's developmental progress.

In many respects, a certain amount of the data collected was retrospective. However, only measured characteristics which were considered reliable over a period of time were used. Similar retrospective biases also applied to the control sample.

Following the interviews the author kept in touch with a variety of outside agencies such as health visitors, social workers and family doctors in order to supplement the data about the families, and especially about the small minority who were unco-operative or reluctant to divulge information. Only the more important factors, however, have been discussed in this book, namely those that were reasonably well defined and had been assessed in a comparatively objective manner. In addition some factors were chosen for discussion because they proved to be closely related to baby battering; others were chosen because they had been cited frequently in the battered baby literature.

The author was fortunate in having had a stable research team available for continuity of assessments and for maintaining the co-operation of the subjects under investigation. Many hours were spent with the psychologist in discussing the choice of factors and methods of measurement that could be used and over the course of the first 15 cases the interview schedules were fully structured. It was not until end of the second year of the study, however, that the goal of obtaining 100 hospitalized battered children was reached. Cases then began to be increasingly referred and this accounts for the excess numbers. Pressure of time and budgetary considerations precluded collecting an equal number of control cases, but the size of the control sample obtained was sufficient for statistical comparisons.

DESCRIPTION OF THE TESTS USED

It was thought expedient to cast the net widely and measure most hypotheses in the literature on a single sample. Information considered important was therefore collected on a wide variety of factors; medical, psychological and social. In order to test the hypotheses certain standardized instruments were selected and *ad hoc* quantifiable measures were constructed (*see* Appendix B). The choice of tests was governed by certain practical considerations. A brief description of each test used in the study is given in the following section.

WECHSLER ADULT INTELLIGENCE SCALE

The test has been widely used in clinical practice and is well standardized. The full scale contains 11 sub-tests covering a wide range of verbal and non-verbal abilities. By detecting discrepancies on different sub-tests the test is useful in confirming the presence of certain psychiatric disturbances. A full WAIS (Wechsler, 1955) takes more than 1 hour to administer. The shortened form used in this study was chosen because a high correlation has been demonstrated between it and the full test. Indeed all possible combinations of four sub-tests of the WAIS (including those used in this study) correlate $r = 0.90$ or higher with full-scale testing (Maxwell, 1957). The ability of battering parents to foresee the consequences of their action is best reflected by the content of the four sub-tests chosen for this study – namely, comprehension, vocabulary, block design and picture arrangement – which are also very good sub-tests of verbal and non-verbal abilities. There are several well recognized methods of arriving at an estimate of a full scale I.Q. (Levy, 1968). The psychologist used one of these methods.

GRIFFITHS DEVELOPMENTAL SCALES

These are designed to test children from 0 to 8 years (Griffiths, 1954,

1967). The test consists of five carefully prepared scales used to measure locomotor, personal–social, hearing–speech, eye–hand and performance skills. The General Quotient (G.Q.) is obtainable by taking the average of all the six sub-quotients. Griffiths (1954) says her purpose in the construction of the scale was

> 'to develop a measuring instrument that shall be at once, reasonably exact, well balanced and comprehensive, so that those activities that later go to make an efficient person, or as many as possible of those skills that are measured in assessing intelligence in older subjects, shall be represented, as it were in embryo, in a valid test of the mentality of a baby'.

Cronbach (1960) reports that the Griffiths Developmental Scale permits more reliable measurement than any other instrument for testing infants' intelligence. The scale's re-test reliability has been shown to be 0.87 (Hindley, 1960).

VINELAND SOCIAL MATURITY SCALE

This scale was used to assess the child's functioning before the injury and to set the scene for the parent to enter more easily into the 'Difficult Times' enquiry. The scale also allowed an assessment of the child's social competence in absentia – for example, if the child had died from his injuries.

The scale provides a definite outline of detailed performances in respect to which children show a progressive capacity for looking after themselves. The items of the scale are arranged in order of increasing average difficulty and represent progressive maturation in the following areas:

Self-help general	Occupation
Self-help eating	Communication
Self-help dressing	Locomotion
Self-direction	Socialization

The definition and method of scoring each item is provided in the Manual of Directions (Doll, 1947). The underlying principles involved in the construction of the scale are similar to those employed in the construction of intelligence tests. Each item is conceived as representing a general growth in social responsibility which is expressed in some detailed performance as an overt expression of that responsibility. The scale provided a particularly convenient measure of assessing individual differences and consequently of extreme deviation in social maturation.

The items of the scale are arranged in order of average age norms and are numbered in arithmetical succession from 1 to 117. They have also been separated in year groups according to the average age scores obtained for the scale as a whole. In this study only the first 61 items, which measure up to the age level of 6 years have been used.

EYSENCK PERSONALITY INVENTORY

Some means of assessing neurotic tendency among the parents was clearly needed in view of the widespread assumption that this was an important factor in baby battering. The Eysenck Personality Inventory (Eysenck and Eysenck, 1964) has been widely used on British samples and provided a measure of an individual's position among the two personality dimensions of neuroticism and extraversion. It takes 5–10 min to complete. According to Eysenck's (1964) theory, persons with a high degree of both neuroticism and extraversion are prone to hysteria, psychopathic and criminal behaviour. Such personality types were thought to constitute an important element of the index population. In describing the extraversion (E) and neuroticism (N) scales on their inventory Eysenck and Eysenck (1964) have stated:

> 'While not wishing to deny the existence and importance of factors additional to E and N, we believe that these two factors contribute more to a description of personality than any other set of two factors outside the cognitive field.'

FOULDS HOSTILITY AND DIRECTION OF HOSTILITY QUESTIONNAIRE

This is a self-administering questionnaire that was chosen because it provided a reliable test of measuring a wide range of aggression, hostility or punitiveness (Caine, Foulds and Hope, 1967). The questionnaire contains five tests of hostility; Acting Out Hostility (AH); Criticism of Others (CO); Paranoid (Projected) Hostility (PH); Self-Criticism (SC); and Guilt (G). Hostility is the sum of all five tests. Direction of Hostility is the sum of the intropunitive tests (with SC counted twice over) less the sum of the extrapunitive tests:

$$\text{Hostility} = AH + CO + PH + SC + G$$
$$\text{Direction of Hostility} = (2\,SC + G) - (AH + CO + PH).$$

Means and Standard Deviations of normal subjects and neurotic and psychotic groups are provided in the manual of Caine, Foulds and Hope (1967).

THE SPIRAL MAZE

Gibson's Spiral Maze (Gibson, 1965) was used to explore the slipshod performance considered characteristic of disturbed individuals. This test is quick and easy to score, and takes only about 2 min to administer. It consists of a spiral path, bordered by heavy black lines which is printed on a large card. Obstacles, represented by the letter O in heavy type, are scattered along the pathway. The subject has to trace round the path with a pencil or ball-point pen, from the centre outwards, in an anti-clockwise direction, and as quickly as he can, but without cutting across the obstacles or touching the edges of the path. The subject's performance is timed with a stop-watch, and he is urged to go as fast as he can. An error score is produced by summing penalty points – example, one for every time the subject's pencil touches the printed lines of the spiral or the obstacles, two for every time the pencil actually penetrates. The error score is adjusted according to the time taken to complete the maze, so that in effect the final score is a rating which compares the subject's accuracy of performance with the average performance of a person of the same age who takes the same length of time.

On this test, well-adjusted persons are both quick and accurate. It was anticipated that high Error scores, indicative of careless performance, would be given by more maladjusted parents. Among the fathers, this proved not to be the case.

GOLDBERG'S GENERAL HEALTH QUESTIONNAIRE

This is a 60-item questionnaire, self-administered and easily scored that provided a reliable method of measuring non-psychotic illness (Goldberg, 1972). It is useful in detecting current emotional disturbance and has been widely used as a screening instrument.

> 'A patient's score on the General Health Questionnaire is in many ways analogous to the erythrocyte sedimentation rate (ESR) in general medicine. In both cases, the high scores merely indicate that there is a high probability that there is something wrong with the patient, but it does not tell the physician the diagnosis. It is an instruction for the physician to examine the patient, and make a diagnosis, using his clinical skills.'
>
> (Goldberg, 1972)

The questionnaire was given at the completion of the psychiatric interview, for it provided a method of validating the author's clinical diagnosis; the probability of a patient with a normal score turning out to be a psychiatric case is fairly low. By comparing the means and standard deviations of scores in the index and control groups, a method of measuring the amount of non-psychotic psychiatric disturbance was obtained.

INTERVIEW SCHEDULES*

In order to ascertain the circumstances which sparked off the battering incident and whether certain factors were operating at the time, a 'Circumstances of Injury' schedule was drawn up. Many questions contained in this schedule were derived from those contained in the University of Rochester Emergency Department Accident Study (Friedman, 1970). In order to achieve maximum objectivity of response, this was placed at the beginning of the medical interview. In contrast to the experience of other researchers in this field, pilot work revealed that it was positively helpful to commence with an enquiry into the child's injury and then branch out into the parent investigation. This method allowed the research team to gain a parent's interest and approach the problem under investigation quite directly.

The 'Psychiatric Interview' schedule was derived from the scheme for case-taking outlined in the text-book of Mayer-Gross, Slater and Roth (1969) and followed a logical sequence, similar to the method of setting out case histories customary in psychiatric clinics. It began with the parents' own origin and health and experiences at school, work and marriage and then went on to the history of the child's birth, infant characteristics, present temperament, behaviour and relations with his parents, and comparison with his siblings. Interpersonal relationships with family, friends and neighbours and family history of mental illness were also covered.

The Social Workers schedule contained two parts. Part 1 was an enquiry into the child-rearing practices used by the parents and included items from the work of Sears, Maccoby and Levin (1957) which applied to the age range of the sample in this study. Only items which came out clearest on his factor analysis were used. The schedule was adopted for fathers with a view to covering similar nurturance-dependence factors in terms of fathers' role. The schedule seemed to lend itself to discussion in the home and was placed at the beginning of the social interview.

Part 2 of the Social Workers schedule was drawn up on the basis of social workers schedules used in other studies (Taylor and Chave,

* Copies of questionnaires used in the study can be obtained from the author.

1964; Chichester Psychiatric Service, 1962). This particularly elaborated upon the extent of the parents' social contacts and allowed for a relatively brief enquiry into economic circumstances and standards in the home.

In the process of analysis, some of the items had to be simplified or omitted. For instance the item about violence between the spouses was often missing because the social worker felt she could not put the question. In addition to her comments on the form itself, the social worker compiled a summary of every case and drew attention to any salient peculiarities or difficulties encountered.

Appendix B

SEMANTIC DIFFERENTIAL

DESCRIPTION OF THE TEST

Following completion of the Vineland Social Maturity Scale parents were asked the questions listed in the Difficult Times Test. (This test and the Semantic Differential form used appear at the end of the appendix and on page 176 (Fig. 40)). On the basis of their responses it was decided whether those questions answered in the affirmative (i.e. categories 2 and 3 for each question) presented a problem to the parent. If more than three problems were mentioned it was decided, by further discussion with the parent, which three were the most severe, as there was insufficient time to explore more than three. Furthermore the exercise of concentrating or applying the same set of self-ratings to different situations becomes difficult. In practice, however, most parents mentioned either no problems or only one or two problems.

For each problem in turn a list of bipolar adjectives derived from the Multiple Affect Adjective Check List (Zuckerman and Lubin, 1965) and in part from the literature related to the battered child syndrome, but adapted to suit the vocabulary of most English subjects, was then presented. The adjective-pairs were:

tense	–	relaxed
enraged	–	calm
understanding	–	resentful
weepy	–	unshaken
rough	–	gentle

affectionate	–	disgusted
cheerful	–	miserable
strong	–	weak
hurt	–	amused
panicky	–	self-controlled
inadequate	–	confident

Instructions were worded around the first problem being dealt with. For example, 'I want you to try and think back to a time or two when . . . has whined and clung to you and prevented you from getting on. Now I'd like you to explain to me by using these descriptions (place Semantic Differential form in front of the subject) what your reactions were. Take the first pair; tense and relaxed. Would . . . 's behaviour make you very tense (point to that extreme) or would you be completely relaxed (point to that extreme) or would you come somewhere in between (point to middle categories).

For some subjects it was not necessary to say more; they grasped the idea at a glance. For others it was better to explain as they went down the list which 'in between' spaces were the ones that best fitted their description and which ones were the best to choose from.

On presentation of a further Semantic Differential form, for a different problem, one had to ensure that the switch to thinking about this problem was maintained as the subject worked through the list of self-ratings. Because the subjects invariably 'thought aloud' as they worked it was relatively easy to carry this checking out.

METHOD OF SCORING AND PRELIMINARY RESULTS FROM PRINCIPAL COMPONENTS ANALYSIS

The number of Semantic Differential forms obtained was 162 for index mothers, 80 for index fathers, 46 for control mothers and 15 for control fathers.

All 242 Semantic Differentials obtained from the index parents were submitted for analyses by the M.R.C. unit's Ingrid 67 programme (Users' Manual kindly provided by Dr. Patrick Slater) so that the 11 self-rating scales might be reduced to a smaller number of factors by means of a principal components analysis.

Self-rating scales had been chosen to include four different clusters; helplessness, lack of self-control, sensitivity and depression. The principal components analysis showed, however, that all 11 scales could best be reduced to a single factor, since the first component accounted for 43 per cent of the variance, while the second accounted for only 13 per cent and the remainder for 7 per cent or less.

On the first component the loadings obtained are shown in Table 32.

Thus, all the self-rating scales were reduced to a single factor of negative affect, which one might call 'Depression'. The three scales loading more than 0.70 on this factor – 'enraged', 'rough', and 'miserable' – suggest a constellation of feelings one might summarize as 'Wretchedness', but since all the negative self-descriptions had high loadings it was decided to label this factor 'Negative Affect'.

Every individual Semantic Differential was now given an approximate factor score by simple summation of scores (1–7) on each of the 11 ratings scales (7 being the score given to each negative pole); hence each Semantic Differential completed could score between 11 and 77.

For some problems very few semantic differentials were obtained.

TABLE 32
Loadings on the First Component of the Principal Components Analysis

Tense	0.67
Enraged	0.74
Resentful	0.66
Weepy	0.53
Rough	0.77
Disgusted	0.64
Miserable	0.79
Weak	0.49
Hurt	0.62
Panicky	0.60
Inadequate	0.68

These were either dropped or, where possible, grouped according to content. In practice all semantic differentials relating to any problem with the child (Questions 1, 2, 3, 4, 5 and 6 on the Difficult Times Text) were treated as all of one kind. Similarly all those problems with the spouse (Questions 3 and 7 on the Difficult Times Test) were treated as of one kind.

Mean factor scores were obtained for the subject-groups; index mothers, index fathers and control mothers for each problem group (problem re child and problem re spouse) separately. Unfortunately there were too few control fathers with these problems to yield reliable means. The means and profiles obtained have been given in Chapter 15. Further detailed work on the principal components analysis is currently being prepared by Mrs. Ruth Hanson.

DIFFICULT TIMES TEST

Case No . . . .

Date . . . .

Place of Interview. . . . .

Given by . . . .

(i) 'Does . . . . sometimes cry (baby) cling (toddler) and prevent you from getting on? Does he keep you awake at night?'

(1) Rarely (2) Sometimes (3) Often

(ii) 'Is . . . . a messy baby, difficult to keep clean? Does he (toddler) throw things around and break things?'

(1) Rarely (2) Sometimes (3) Often

(iii) 'Is your husband able to help with . . . . as much as-you would like? Does he have long working hours, days away, evenings out?' (Mothers) or 'Does your wife cope with the baby and the home all right?' (Fathers)

(1) Rarely (2) Sometimes (3) Often

(iv) 'Does . . . . . often have a temper tantrum (toddler) or not stop screaming (baby) because he can't get his own way?' 'Is it a problem to you?'

(1) Rarely (2) Sometimes (3) Often

(v) 'Does . . . . . ever absolutely refuse to do something you want him to? (toddler). Refuse to take his food? (baby)'

(1) Rarely (2) Sometimes (3) Often

(vi) 'Those are the more common problems in bringing up children, but have you any other difficulties with . . . . . apart from the ones I have mentioned?'

(1) Rarely (2) Sometimes (3) Often
Specify Problem . . . .

. . . .

(vii) 'Just before . . . . came into hospital, were there any particular difficulties between you and your husband/wife?'

(1) Rarely (2) Sometimes (3) Often

Specify Problem . . . .

. . . .

(viii) 'Just before . . . came into hospital, were there any particular difficulties between you and your relatives or other members of your family?'

(1) Rarely (2) Sometimes (3) Often

Specify Problem . . . .

. . . .

(ix) 'Do you have difficulties with your other children?'

(1) Rarely (2) Sometimes (3) Often

Specify Problem . . . .

. . . .

(x) 'Do you have any difficulties with other people such as neighbours and friends?'

(1) Rarely (2) Sometimes (3) Often

Specify Problem . . . .

. . . .

Appendix C

METHOD OF ADJUSTING FOR SOCIAL CLASS

Social class and the cultural background it broadly represents have been shown to have some degree of association with most psychological variables (Sears, Maccoby and Levin, 1957; Newson and Newson, 1963). Because such a high proportion of the index sample were of low social class it was not possible – while controlling for other important factors – to obtain a control sample of equally low social class (Table 33 shows the social class distribution of index and controls). To resolve this problem a method of weighting, used by Newson (1973a), has been adopted. Four examples are given below.

TABLE 33
Social Class Distribution Among Index and Control Groups

	I	*II*	*III*	*IV*	*V*
Index group (per cent)	0 (0)	3 (3)	26 (22)	56 (48)	33 (28)
Control group (per cent)	5 (10)	4 (8)	26 (50)	14 (27)	3 (6)

$\chi^2 = 26.29$, d.f. = 1; $p < 0.001$ (for non-manual vs manual)

EXAMPLE 1. 'NOT VERY DEMONSTRATIVE'

Table 34 shows the proportion of index and controls rated as not very demonstrative towards their child within each social class and for each sample as a whole. The procedure for adjusting the index sample to represent the social class distribution of the controls is as follows.

(*i*) Take the percentage of control cases in each social class and multiply by the percentage of index cases who were not very demonstrative – for example 50 per cent of the controls were in social class III. Multiply this percentage by the percentage of index cases in social class III who were not very demonstrative – for example 50 per cent by 38 per cent, giving 19 per cent, (this appears in the second line of Table 34 as class adjusted per cent). This procedure is carried out for each social class in turn.

(*ii*) Add the class adjusted percentages in each social class to give an overall percentage for the index sample adjusted for social class (Adjusted Total). Convert this percentage into numbers based on the total for the index sample – for example 38 per cent is converted into a new raw total based on 105 and becomes $n = 40$. This appears as 40/105.

(*iii*) Comparing the total for the control sample (6/50 in the table) with adjusted total for the index sample 40/105 calculate χ^2 and level of significance.

(*iv*) Compare χ^2 between the index and control groups before and after adjusting for social class (both χ^2 values are given below the table). It will be seen that for this particular variable χ^2 before social class adjustment was 18.40 ($p < 0.001$) and after social class adjustment χ^2 was 9.83 ($p < 0.01$). Therefore, in the text of the results this is recorded as: 'This finding remained significant after class control'.

EXAMPLE 2. 'NOT MUCH TIME TO PLAY'

Table 35 shows an example of a variable where the contrast between index and controls became insignificant after adjustments were made for social class. In the text of the results this is recorded as 'This finding became insignificant when adjusted for social class', or, 'insignificant after class control'.

EXAMPLE 3. NEUROSIS

Table 36 shows the social class breakdowns for psychiatric diagnosis of neurosis – variables which might be regarded as particularly open to bias. It will be seen that there is an association between diagnosis and social class which may or may not have been due to bias; despite this the difference between index and controls remained highly significant.

TABLE 34

Social Class Distribution Among Index and Control Mothers who were 'Not Very Demonstrative' before* and after† Adjustments for Social Class.

	I	*II*	*III*	*IV*	*V*	*Total*	*Adjusted total*
Index (per cent)	0 (0)	1 (33)	9 (38)	23(43)	16 (61)	50/105 (48)	40/105
Class adjusted (per cent)	0	3	19	12	4		38
Control(per cent)	2 (50)	1 (25)	2 (8)	0(0)	1 (50)		

* $\chi^2 = 18.40$; d.f. = 1; $p < 0.001$
† $\chi^2 = 9.83$; d.f. = 1; $p < 0.01$

TABLE 35

Social Class Distribution Among Index and Control Mothers on 'Not Much Time to Play' before* and after† Adjustments for Social Class

	I	*II*	*III*	*IV*	*V*	*Total*	*Adjusted total*
Index (per cent)	0 (0)	1 (33)	10 (43)	28 (53)	13 (50)	52/105 (50)	44/105
Class adjusted (per cent)	0	3	22	14	3		42
Control (per cent)	0 (0)	1 (25)	5 (19)	6 (43)	1 (50)	13/50 (26)	

* $\chi^2 = 6.19$; d.f. = 1; $p < 0.05$
† $\chi^2 = 3.03$; d.f. = 1; N.S.

TABLE 36
Social Class Distribution Among Index and Control Mothers on Neurosis, before* and after† Adjustments for Social Class

	I	*II*	*III*	*IV*	*V*	*Total*	*Adjusted total*
Index (per cent)	0 (0)	1 (33)	11 (46)	24 (45)	17 (61)	53/108 (50)	45/108
Class adjusted (per cent)	0	3	23	12	4		42
Control (per cent)	1 (25)	0 (0)	1 (4)	3 (21)	0 (0)	5/49 (10)	

* $\chi^2 = 12.08$; d.f. = 1; $p < 0.001$ † $\chi^2 = 14.13$; d.f. = 1; $p < 0.001$

TABLE 37
Social Class Distribution Among Index and Control Fathers on Psychopathy before* and after† Adjustments for Social Class

	I	*II*	*III*	*IV*	*V*	*Total*	*Adjusted total*
Index (per cent)	0 (0)	0 (0)	9 (45)	12 (32)	11 (46)	32/84 (38)	29/84
Class adjusted (per cent)	0	0	23	9	3		35
Control (per cent)	0 (0)	0 (0)	0 (0)	0 (0)	0 (0)	0/22 (0)	

* $\chi^2 = 10.38$; d.f. = 1; $p < 0.001$ † $\chi^2 = 8.79$; d.f. = 1; $p < 0.01$

TABLE 38
Social Class Distribution Among Index and Controls on 'Pre-Marital Conception' before* and after† Adjustments for Social Class

	I	*II*	*III*	*IV*	*V*	*Total*	*Adjusted total*
Index (per cent)	0 (0)	0 (0)	17 (71)	38 (71)	20 (71)	75/107 (71)	64/107
Class adjusted (per cent)	0	0	36	20	4	60	60
Control (per cent)	1 (25)	1 (25)	8 (31)	6 (43)	0 (0)	16/49 (33)	

EXAMPLE 4. PSYCHOPATHY

Table 37 shows the social class breakdown for psychopathy among the fathers. This may or may not be class-linked but is rare in a general population and not surprisingly, therefore, non-existent in the controls. Adjusting the index findings for social class reduced the χ^2 but the finding nevertheless remained significant.

EXAMPLE 5. PRE-MARITAL CONCEPTION

Table 38 shows the social class breakdown for index and control samples on pre-marital conception. This is an example of a variable that is only slightly class-linked; and this is shown by the distribution for index and control samples. (Among the controls this is not as obvious because the numbers are small.) Though the χ^2 value diminished after social class control it remained definitely significant.

Appendix D

QUESTIONS AND RESPONSE CATEGORIES AND CATEGORY COMBINATIONS FOR χ^2 TEST

Questions and response categories	*Category combinations for* χ^2 *test*
Social class This was based on the Registrar General's Classification of Occupations, 1966.	
*Pre-marital pregnancy was questioned and checked on the basis of dates of marriage and birth of first child.	
Attitude to pregnancy 'Did you feel when you were expecting . . that it was a good time to have a baby? Or would it have been better to wait?' (*a*) delighted; (*b*) pleased on the whole, some reservations; (*c*) displeased.	*a* and *b* vs *c* also *a* vs *b* and *c*
**Abortion* 'Would you have liked an abortion when pregnant with . . ?' No/Yes	
**Contraception* 'Do you want any more children?' 'Are you doing anything about contraception?' No/Yes	

Questions and response categories	*Category combinations for* χ^2 *test*
Husband's reaction to relevant pregnancy 'How did your husband feel about your pregnancy with . . ?' *or* if not the biological father 'How did your husband take to . . ?' (*a*) delighted; (*b*) pleased on the whole; (*c*) generally displeased.	*a* vs *b* and *c* (= ambivalent) also *a* and *b* vs *c*
Evaluation of partner 'How much alike do you think you and your husband are? Would you rather have . . to grow up to be like you or like your husband?' (*a*) thinks highly of; (*b*) appreciates on the whole, dislikes some things; (*c*) thinks poorly of.	*a* and *b* vs *c*
Partners relationship with child 'Will you tell me how . . . 's father gets on with him? Does he help with . . . ?' (*a*) very fond of child, enjoys playing etc.; (*b*) quite fond of child, takes interest; (*c*) rejects or is not interested in the child.	*a* and *b* vs *c*
Agreement on child-rearing practices 'In general, how well would you say you and your husband agree about the best way to handle . . . ?' (*a*) discuss and/or usually agree; (*b*) disagree frequently; (*c*) partner doesn't participate.	*a* vs *b* and *c* also *a* and *b* vs *c*
Head of household 'Who makes the important decisions for the family?' (*a*) father; (*b*) share; (*c*) mother	*a* and *b* vs *c*
Personal significance of religion 'Does religion mean anything to you?' (*a*) nothing; (*b*) goes to or nominally attached to place of worship; (*c*) personal faith.	*a* and *b* vs *c*

Items marked * are from psychiatric interview.
Items marked † are 'Difficult Times' test questions.
Unmarked Items are from social worker's Home Visit Schedule.

Questions and response categories	*Category combinations for χ^2 test*
Religious background (*a*) none; (*b*) one or both parents nominally religious; (*c*) one or both parents had personal faith.	*a* vs *b* and *c*
Amenities (*a*) fixed bath (own or shared); (*b*) running water inside own accomodation; (*c*) W.C. indoors; (*d*) own kitchen.	all present vs, one or more missing
Child's sleeping arrangements (*a*) own room; (*b*) shares room with sibs; (*c*) shares bed with sibs; (*d*) shares room with parents; (*e*) shares bed with parents.	*a* vs others for 'lacks own room' also *a* and *b* vs others for 'cramped sleeping accommodation.'
M.S.W.'s assessment of housing (*a*) good; (*b*) reasonable condition; (*c*) dilapidated.	*a* and *b* vs *c*
M.S.W.'s assessment of care of home (*a*) obsessionally clean and tidy; (*b*) reasonable; (*c*) dirty and untidy.	*a* and *b* vs *c*
Contact with (i) parents (ii) other relatives (iii) neighbours (iv) friends (*a*) almost daily; (*b*) approximately weekly; (*c*) monthly; (*d*) infrequently; (*e*) never.	*a*, *b* and *c* vs *d* and *e*
Regular social activities (*a*) sports; (*b*) other clubs; (*c*) evening classes; (*d*) public house; (*e*) church; (*f*) visiting friends; (*g*) others	any vs none

Questions and response categories	*Category combinations for χ^2 tests*
Opportunity for breaks from care of child 'Can . . . play (or be in pram) out of doors without you being with him all the time? Can baby sitting be arranged?'	Yes to one or both vs no to both and including cases where baby sitting 'available' but not required
Assessment of allowance (*a*) generous; (*b*) adequate; (*c*) inadequate	*a* and *b* vs *c*
Any significant worries 'Are any of the following worries for you?' (*a*) money; (*b*) domestic friction; (*c*) own health; (*d*) health of others; (*e*) housing; (*f*) employment; (*g*) marital status; (*h*) moral or personal.	none or one vs two or more
Reaction to total situation 'How satisfied are you with your present life?' (*a*) very; (*b*) fairly; (*c*) not at all.	*a* vs *b* and *c*
Physical punishment ' How often do you spank (or smack) . . . ?' (*a*) frequently and severely; (*b*) slaps fairly often, occasionally spanks; (*c*) occasionally; (*d*) never.	*a* and *b* vs *c* and *d*
Withholding love 'What do you say to . . when he's been naughty?' (*a*) Doesn't love him, he's a bad child; (*b*) tells him he's been naughty; (*c*) ignores.	*a* vs *b* and *c*
Deprivation of privileges 'Do you ever deprive . . . of something as a way of disciplining him? How often do you do this?' (*a*) frequently; (*b*) sometimes; (*c*) rarely	*a* vs *b* and *c*

Questions and response categories	*Category combinations for χ^2 test*
Material rewards 'Do you have any system of rewarding . . for being good?' (*a*) rarely uses material rewards; (*b*) sometimes; (*c*) often.	*a* vs *b* and *c*
Verbal encouragement 'Do you tell . . . he's been good?' (*a*) rarely; (*b*) sometimes; (*c*) readily.	*a* vs *b* and *c*
Age at bowel training 'When did you start putting . . . on the potty?' (*a*) under 6 months; (*b*) under 12 months; (*c*) under 18 months; (*d*) under 24 months; (*e*) 24 months and over.	*a* and *b* vs *c*, *d* and *e*
Severity of training 'When do you expect . . . to stop wearing nappies (baby)? How do you try and teach him to be dry? What do you do when he has an accident? (toddler)' (*a*) child left on potty for lengthy periods, punishes accidents (*b*) some toileting, moderate disapproval for accidents; (*c*) child more or less trains self, no scolding.	*a* vs *b* and *c*
Restrictions 'How important do you think it is (or will be) for . . to be careful about marking walls and jumping on the furniture?' (*a*) very restrictive; (*b*) moderately restrictive; (*c*) no restrictions	*a* and *b* vs *c*
Surveillance 'Do you keep track of (toddler) or can you leave him on his own quite a bit? How often do you go and see how (baby) is?' (*a*) checks frequently; (*b*) checks fairly often; (*c*) practically never checks.	*a* vs *b* and *c*

Questions and response categories	*Category combinations for χ^2 test*
Standards of obedience 'Some parents expect their children to obey immediately when they tell them to be quiet or pick something up. Others don't think it is terribly important for the child to obey right away. How do you feel about this?' (*a*) generally expect child to obey on first or second demand; (*b*) wants child to obey but expects some delay; (*c*) does not expect obedience.	*a* and *b* vs *c* also *a* vs *b* and *c*
'Does . . ever absolutely refuse to do something you want him to do (toddler)?' 'Refuse to take his food (baby)?' 'Is it a problem to you?' (*a*) rarely does; (*b*) sometimes or often does but no problem; (*c*) sometimes or often does; a problem to the mother.	*a* and *b* vs *c*
†'Does . . . sometimes cry (baby) cling (toddler) and prevent you from getting on? Does he keep you awake at night?' as above	
†'Is . . . a messy baby, difficult to keep clean? Does he (toddler) throw things around and break things?' as above	
†'Is your husband able to help with . . as much as you would like? Does he have long working hours, days away, evenings out?' (Mothers) *or* 'Does your wife cope with the baby at home all right?' (Fathers)† Yes/No	
Mother's responsiveness to crying 'All babies cry, of course. Some mothers feel that if you pick a baby up every time it cries you will spoil it. Others think you should never let a baby cry for very long. How do you (did you) feel about this?' (*a*) unresponsive; (*b*) 'it depends'; (*c*) invariably picks up.	*a* and *b* vs *c* also *a* vs *b* and *c* also *b* vs *a* and *c*

Questions and response categories	*Category combinations for* χ^2 *test*
Punishment for screaming 'When . . . screams in temper, not in pain – what do you do?' (*a*) screams back, slaps; (*b*) puts out of earshot for time; (*c*) never punishes.	*a* and *b* vs *c* *b* vs *a* and *c*
Punishment for aggression towards parents 'How do you handle . . when he hits you?' (*a*) severe punishment; (*b*) moderate punishment; (*c*) no punishment.	*a* and *b* vs *c*
Duration of breast feeding 'Could you tell me something about how breast feeding went in the early stages? For how long was . . . breast fed? Why not? Any other reason?' (*a*) not for psychological reasons; (*b*) not for physical reasons; (*c*) for up to 1 month; (*d*) for up to 3 months (*e*) over 3 months.	*a* and *b* vs *c*, *d* and *e*
Schedule of feeding 'There has been a lot of talk about whether it is better to have a regular feeding schedule for a baby, or to feed him whenever he is hungry. How do you feel about this? How do you handle this with . . . ?' (*a*) rigid feeding schedule; (*b*) rough feeding schedule; (*c*) complete self-demand.	*a* vs *b* and *c*
Encouragement of good feeding 'Have you any problems about . . . eating what or how he should? What do you do about it? What do you do when he eats well?' (*a*) doesn't bother what child eats; (*b*) shows pleasure when child eats well; (*c*) is very emotional over feeding.	*a* and *b* vs *c*

Questions and response categories	*Category combinations for X^2 test*
Enjoyment of child 'What sort of thing do you enjoy in . . . ? Do you get much pleasure out of caring for him . . . or do you think he'll be more interesting when he's older?' (*a*) doesn't enjoy; (*b*) enjoys; (*c*) child is 'her life'.	*b* vs *a* and *c* also *a* and *b* vs *c* also *a* vs *b* and *c*
Time to play 'Do you have time to spend with your child besides the time that is necessary for feeding and changing him.' (*a*) never; (*b*) sometimes; (*c*) often.	*a* and *b* vs *c*
Affectionate demonstrativeness 'Tel me what you do in the time you spend with your child? Do you cuddle or sing to . . . ?' (*a*) not an affectionate type of mother; (*b*) moderately warm; (*c*) very warm.	*a* and *b* vs *c*
Childhood experience of warmth from mother 'Did your own mother have a lot of time to spend with you when you were small? Did she seem warm and affectionate?' (*a*) own mother/caretaker not demonstrative; (*b*) did show affection often; (*c*) very warm.	*a* vs *b* and *c*
Childhood experience of discipline 'How would you describe your mother's (repeat question for fathers) attitude towards you? Was she (he) (*a*) normal?; (*b*) strict?; (*c*) rejecting?; (*d*) harsh?'	*a* vs *b* *c* and *d* also *a* and *b*, vs *c* and *d*

Glossary

AGITATED DEPRESSION

A state of restlessness, usually arising out of subjective feelings of apprehension and accompanied by an inability to relax or to concentrate and associated with depression.

ALLERGIC RHINITIS

Inflammation of the nasal mucous membranes which may be caused by an allergen. Frequently called hay fever.

ALVEOLAR

Pertaining to the bony socket of a tooth.

AMENORRHOEA

Absence of menstruation.

ANOREXIA NERVOSA

A condition more common in females, characterized by a morbid aversion to food, with serious weight loss and a fear of regaining normal weight. Amenorrhoea, the appearance of lanugo hair and a variety of biochemical disorders also occur.

CALLUS

New growth of incompletely organized bony tissue that is part of the reparative process and surrounds the bone ends of a fracture.

CEREBRAL PALSY

Paralysis due to injury of the brain

CHI-SQUARE χ^2

A test of statistical significance used to determine whether the differences observed in a population are likely or unlikely to be the result of chance.

CLAVICLE

The collar bone.

COELIAC SYNDROME

A syndrome in which intestinal malabsorption of fat results in bulky, loose, foul smelling stools. Failure to gain weight, anorexia, weakness and consequent vitamin deficiencies with their accompanying symptoms result.

CONGENITAL DEFECT

A defect existing from birth.

CONGENITAL INDIFFERENCE TO PAIN

These children, like those with a neurogenic sensory deficit (q.v.) fail to react normally to body injury and skeletal changes are the same as those seen in battered children. An uncommon condition but an important one to exclude before making the diagnosis of 'inadequately explained injuries'.

CONGENITAL SPHEROCYSTOSIS

A chronic disorder of the blood-forming system existing from birth, that results in red blood cells that are spherical rather than biconcave in shape causing them to readily break up.

CORRELATION COEFFICIENT

The degree of association between two characteristics in a series of observations. If the value of the correlation coefficient is 0 or close to it, the characteristics are not interrelated: if close to +1 there is a close association between them; if near −1, an inverse relationship, i.e. as one value increases the other decreases to an equivalent degree.

CORTICAL

The outer part of the bone.

DEVELOPMENT QUOTIENT (D.Q.)

The mathematical expression of the relation between developmental age and actual or chronological age:

$$DQ = \frac{\text{development age}}{\text{actual or chronological age}}$$

DIAPHYSIS

The shaft of a long bone.

ECLECTIC

A system of medicine in which the psychiatrist selects from various schools what he considers to be the best methods of treatment.

EHLERS–DANLOS SYNDROME

A collection of symptoms and signs that includes hyperelastic skin, hyperflexible joints, fragile skin and blood vessels and subcutaneous nodules.

ELECTROENCEPHALOGRAM (EEG)

A graphic record of the minute changes in electric potential associated with the activity of the cerebral cortex, as detected by electrodes applied to the surface of the scalp.

ENCEPHALOCELE

Hernia of the brain through a congenital or traumatic opening of the skull.

EPIGASTRIC

Part of the abdomen immediately over the stomach.

EPIPHYSIS

A portion of bone attached for a time to a bone by cartilage, but subsequently becomes consolidated with the principal bone.

ESR (ERYTHROCYTE SEDIMENTATION RATE)

The rate at which red cells settle out of citrated blood. Increase in sedimentation rate occurs in a number of pathological states.

EXUDATES

The material that has passed through the walls of vessels into adjacent tissues or spaces in inflammation.

FATIGUE FRACTURE (STRESS FRACTURE)

A break in the metatarsal bones or fibula without obvious trauma.

FEMUR

The thigh bone.

FIBULA

The slender bone at the outer part of the leg, that lies adjacent to the tibia (q.v.).

GROUP PSYCHOTHERAPY

Any form of psychotherapy (q.v.) in which several persons are treated simultaneously usually by one psychotherapist.

HAEMATOMA

A focalized extravasation of blood (resulting from rupture of blood vessels) which soon clots to form a solid mass and readily becomes encapsulated by connective tissue.

HEMIPARESIS

Paralysis of one side of the body.

HIRSCHPRUNG'S DISEASE

Congenital dilatation of the colon.

HYDROCEPHALUS

An increase in the volume of cerebrospinal fluid within the skull.

HYPERNATREMIA

Abnormally high sodium level in the blood which can cause loss of body water resulting in dehydration.

HYSTERICAL PERSONALITY

A type of character structure that is shallow, narcissistic and egocentric. Such individuals are unable to make deep and enduring relationships with others and have a tendency to confuse fantasy with fact.

INCIDENCE

The number of cases of a disease appearing per unit of population within a defined time interval.

INFANTICIDE

A woman who deliberately causes the death of her child under the age of 12 months is found guilty of infanticide instead of murder if the jury is satisfied that the balance of her mind was disturbed by the birth and subsequent lactation. She is then dealt with as if she had committed manslaughter.

INFANTILE CORTICAL HYPEROSTOSIS (CAFFEY'S SYNDROME)

A condition of unknown aetiology occurring in infants, characterized by irritability associated with the appearance of tender swellings of soft tissues which overlie bones of the extremities, followed by x-ray signs of hypertrophy of bony tissue.

INFANTILE SPASMS

These consist of periodic spells of jack-knife (whole body) flexions or extensions and mental retardation. The EEG shows chaotic abnormality (hypsarrhythmia).

INFANTILISM

The persistence of infantile or childish traits and characteristics into adolescent and adult life.

INTELLIGENCE QUOTIENT (I.Q.)

A figure used to designate a person's intelligence which can be arrived at by dividing the mental age by the chronological age.

INTRACRANIAL HAEMORRHAGE

Bleeding that has occurred within the skull.

LESION

The alteration, structural or functional, due to injury.

LITTLE LEAGUE ELBOW

A manifestation of repetitive injury whereby the vigorous mechanical activity of throwing a ball causes incomplete avulsions (ephiphyseal separations) around the region of the elbow. The resulting change may simulate those of battered children but the age of the patient is appreciably older.

MARASMUS

A gradual wasting of the tissues of the body from an insufficient food supply.

MEAN

The arithmetic mean or average is calculated by adding the individual values of a series and dividing the result by the number of observations.

MESENTERY

A fold of the peritoneum that connects the intestine with the posterior abdominal wall.

METAPHYSIS

The region of growth between the epiphysis (q.v.) and diaphysis (q.v.) of a bone. Also called the epiphyseal plate.

MINIMAL BRAIN DYSFUNCTION – (MINIMAL BRAIN DAMAGE, HYPERKINESIS, 'CLUMSY CHILDREN')

A term applied to children of normal intelligence who have certain behavioural or learning disabilities which are presumed to be associated with faulty function of the central nervous system. The deviations appear in various combinations of impairment of perception, behaviour, language, attention span, and motor function (of which hyperactivity is just one deviation). The term is not a diagnosis but is made up of a heterogenous mass of different problems which require full assessment.

MODE

The value in a series of observations which occurs most frequently.

MUCOSA

A mucous membrane.

NEUROGENIC SENSORY DEFICIT

A sensory deficiency occurring as a result of such conditions as paraplegia or meningomyelocele that may result in separation of epiphyses in the lower extremities following physiotherapy or other injury. The severity of the injury may not be appreciated and the x-ray changes are indistinguishable from those of the battered child.

NEUROSIS – (ALSO CALLED PSYCHONEUROSIS)

A group of reactions characterized chiefly by anxiety, which may be directly felt and expressed or unconsciously controlled. In contrast to psychotic disorders (q.v.) there is no gross disorganization of personality in relation to external reality. Individuals suffering from psychoneurotic disorders usually present a history of unusual difficulties in development related to special stresses or deprivations in early life which influence the form of the disorders in terms of symptoms and susceptibilities.

OBSESSION

An idea or emotion that persists in an individual's mind in spite of any conscious attempts to remove it.

OBSESSIVE-COMPULSIVE PERSONALITY

One characterized by chronic, excessive or obsessive (q.v.) concern with adherence to standards of conscience or conformity resulting in inhibited, rigid, overtly conscientious behaviour.

OPTIC ATROPHY

Degeneration of the optic nerve.

OSTEOGENESIS IMPERFECTA

A defect of bone formation and calcification of unknown cause but often hereditary or familial, characterized by bone fragility and blue sclerae. The first of many fractures may occur at or before birth, in infancy or later in childhood.

OSTEOID OSTEOMA

A small benign tumour of bone, occurring almost exclusively in younger age groups and characteristically accompanied by severe pain.

PAPILLOEDEMA

Oedema or swelling of the optic nerve.

PATHOGNOMONIC

Characteristic of a disease.

PERINEUM

The region between the anus and the scrotum in the male; between the anus and vulva in the female.

PERIOSTEUM

The vascular fibrous membrane covering the surface of a bone.

PERIPHERAL CHOROIDRETINAL ATROPHY

Degeneration of the peripheral parts of the choroid (the vascular tunic of the eye lying between the sclera and the retina) and the retina (the light receptive layer of the eye).

PERITONITIS

Inflammation of the serous membrane lining the interior of the abdominal cavity and viscera.

PERPHENAZINE – (CHLORPHENAZINE, FENTAZIN)

A major tranquilizer and phenothiazine derivative, that has actions and uses similar to those of chlorpromazine. Side-effects include drowsiness and extra-pyramidal symptoms.

PERSONALITY DISORDERS

A group of disorders characterized by patholigical trends in personality structure, with minimal subjective anxiety, manifested in most instances, by a life-long pattern of abnormal action or behaviour, rather than mental or emotional symptoms.

PETECHIAL

A description of minute, rounded spots of haemorrhage on a surface such as skin, mucous membrane or on a cross-sectional surface of an organ.

POST-PARTUM DEPRESSION

Two or three days after a confinement many women undergo a brief episode of depression and tearfulness known as 'post-natal blues' – regarded as a 'normal' phenomenon. Frank psychotic illness however is at least four times as common in the puerperium as in pregnancy and hormonal, personality and environmental factors contribute. Depressive symptoms are common and do not differ from neurotic reactions (q.v.) generally; childbirth and its consequences act as both a physical and a mental stress, liable to provoke neurotic symptoms in susceptible personalities.

POSTERIOR SUBCAPSULAR CATARACT

Opacity beneath the posterior part of the capsule of the lens within the eye.

PRE-RETINAL HAEMORRHAGE

Bleeding that occurs anterior to the internal limiting membrane of the retina.

PREVALENCE

The number of cases of a disease existing in a population at any given time.

PROXIMAL

Situated towards the point of attachment or the centre of a body.

PSEUDOCYST

A saclike space containing liquid, semiliquid or gas but without a definite lining membrane.

PSYCHOMOTOR EQUIVALENT

A twilight state, particularly associated with temporal lobe epilepsy in which the patient may exhibit acute psychotic symptoms, delusional ideas, hallucinations, compulsive acts and other phenomena for which he is not aware. There may be amnesia following the attacks.

PSYCHOPATH (SEE P. 110–111)†

One characterized by emotional immaturity with marked defects of judgement, prone to impulsive behaviour without considerations of others and without evidence of learning by experience.

PSYCHOPATHOLOGY

The pathology of mental disease. Its theme is the whole man in illness, in so far as the illness reveals itself in the psychic sphere and is psychologically conditioned.

PSYCHOTHERAPY

A method of treating illness based on the use of psychological rather than physical techniques. It varies in complexity from the simplest supportive psychotherapy, aimed at aiding the patient to overcome immediate difficulties by guidance, environmental manipulation, reassurance and persuasion to the more complex psychoanalytically-orientated psychotherapies such as psychoanalysis based on the work of Freud. Behaviour therapies such as operant or 'positive' conditioning are included.

PSYCHOTIC

The reaction of an individual to external stress or injury, characterized generally by severe mood disturbance, profound introspection and withdrawal from reality, with failure to test and evaluate external reality adequately, formation of delusions or hallucinations and regression presenting the appearance of personality disintegration. Included in the grouping of psychotic disorders are schizophrenic (q.v.), affective, and paranoid reactions.

PURPURIC

A description of haemorrhages occurring in the skin, mucous membranes and elsewhere.

RADIUS

The outer of the two bones of the forearm.

RECIDIVIST

A confirmed, relapsed or habitual criminal.

RETINAL DETACHMENT

Separation of the retina (or light receptive layer) from the choroid (vascular membrane between the retina and the outer fibrous coating of the eye).

ROENTGEN

An alternative term of x-ray:- Named after William Röntgen who discovered x-rays in 1895 and laid the foundation for the sciences of roentgenology and radiology.

ROLE REVERSAL

A reversal of the dependency role in which parents turn to their infants and small children for nurturing and protection. Two basic elements are postulated to be involved – a high expectation and demand by the parent for the infant's performance and a corresponding parental disregard of the infant's own needs, limited abilities and helplessness.

SCAPULA

The shoulder blade, the large flat, triangular bone forming the back of the shoulder.

SCHIZOID PERSONALITY

One given to seclusiveness, emotional rigidity, introversion and unsocial behaviour.

SCHIZOPHRENIA

One of a group of psychotic reactions, often beginning after adolescence or in young adulthood, characterized by fundamental disturbances in reality relationships and concept formations, with associated mood, behavioural and intellectual disturbances in varying degrees and mixtures. These reactions are marked by a tendency to withdraw from reality, inappropriate mood, unpredictable disturbances in stream of thought, regressive tendencies to the point of deterioration and often hallucinations and delusions.

In *paranoid schizophrenia,* delusions of persecution or of grandeur or both, hallucinations and ideas of reference predominate, and sometimes are systematized. The patient is often more intact and less bizarre in other areas, but generally is hostile, grandiose, excessively religious, and sometimes hypochondriacal.

SCURVY

A nutritional disorder caused by deficiency of vitamin C and characterized by extreme weakness, spongy gums and a tendency to develop haemorrhages under the skin, and peritoneum.

SKELETAL SURVEY

X-raying of the total skeleton.

SPINA BIFIDA

A complete or incomplete congenital cleft of the vertebral column.

STANDARD DEVIATION

The statistical expression of a group of observations must give not only the average (*mean*, (q.v.)) but also the extent of the scatter about the average. The 'standard deviation' (S.D.) expresses the variation. In a normal distribution curve, 95 per cent of the observations are covered by the mean ± 2 S.D.s.

STATISTICAL SIGNIFICANCE

Statistical analyses are designed to determine the degree of chance between two groups of observations being related. This degree of probability is expressed as a percentage. A difference is said to be 'significant' if the probability is less than 5 per cent i.e. there is less than 1 chance in 20 that this could have occurred by chance. A more accurate representation of the 'significance' of differences is expressed by giving the probability as a value e.g. $0.01 > 0.001$ i.e. it lies between 1 in 100 and 1 in 1000 (*see also* Chi-square).

SUBARACHNOID HAEMORRHAGE

A collection of blood beneath the arachnoid membrane (a covering of the brain).

SUBDURAL HAEMATOMA

A collection of blood beneath the dura mater (the outer covering of the brain).

SUBGALEAL HAEMATOMA

A collection of blood beneath the galea aponeurotica (a fibrous sheath beneath the muscle connecting the eyebrows with the back of the skull).

SUBPERIOSTEAL HAEMORRHAGE

Bleeding beneath the periosteum (q.v.)

SYNDROME

A group of symptoms and signs, which when considered together characterize a disease or lesion.

SYPHILIS

A prenatal or acquired chronic systemic infection, most often contracted in sexual intercourse. Lesions may occur in every tissue or vascular organ of the body and the disease may give rise to symptoms characteristic of other diseases. Hence syphilis is called the 'great imitator'.

TIBIA

The larger of the two bones of the leg, commonly called the shin bone.

TRAUMA

A form of injury caused by any physical agent.

ULNA

The bone on the inner side of the forearm, articulating with the humerus and the head of the radius above, and with the radius below.

WHIPLASH INJURY

A sudden movement of the head causing it to be thrown backwards and on recoil to be pitched forward. The movement may be violent because the restraining muscles of the neck are relaxed.

References

The Abused Child (1963). Principles and suggested language for legislation on reporting of the physically abused child. U.S. Department of Health, Education and Welfare, Welfare Administration. Children's Bureau, Washington, D.C. Government Printing Office

Adelson, L. (1961). 'Slaughter of the innocents: a study of forty-six homicides in which the victims were children.' *New Engl. J. Med.* **264**, 1345–1349

Adelson, L. (1963). 'Homicide by starvation: the nutritional variant of the "battered child". *J. Am. Med. Ass.* **186**, 104–106

Adler, A. (1951). *The Practice and Theory of Individual Psychology*, (Translated by P. Radin). New York: Humanities Press

Allen, A. and Morton, A. (1961). *This is Your Child. The Story of the National Society for the Prevention of Cruelty to Children.* London: Routledge and Kegan Paul

Allen, H. D., Ten Bensel, R. W. and Raile, R. B. (1968). 'The battered child syndrome – II. Social and psychiatric aspects.' *Minn. Med.* **52**, 155–156

Altman, D. H. and Smith, R. L. (1960). 'Unrecognized trauma in infants and children.' *J. Bone J Surg.* **42**, 407–413

American Academy of Pediatrics (1966). 'Committee on infant and pre-school child. Maltreatment of children: The physically abused child.' *Pediatrics* **37**, 377–382

American Humane Association (1963). *Guidelines for Legislation to Protect the Battered Child: Basic Principles and Concepts.* Denver, Colorado, Children's Division

American Humane Association (1966). *Child Abuse Legislation.* Denver, Colorado, Children's Division

American Psychiatric Association (1952). *Diagnostic and Statistical Manual for Mental Disorders.* Washington, D.C.A.P.A.

Aptekar, J. (1931). *Anjea: Infanticide, Abortion and Contraception in Savage Society.* New York: William Godwin

Ariès, P. (1962). *Centuries of Childhood.* Harmondsworth, Middlesex, England: Penguin Books

Astley, R. (1953). 'Multiple metaphyseal fractures in small children.' *Br. J. Radiol.* **26**, 577–583

Bain, K. (1963). 'The physically abused child.' *Pediatrics* **31**, 895–897

Bakan, D. (1971). *Slaughter of the Innocents: A Study of the Battered Child Phenomenon.* San Francisco: Jossey-Bass

Bakwin, H (1952). 'Roentgenographic changes in the bones following trauma in infants.' *J. Newark Beth Israel Hosp.* **3**, 17

Bakwin, H. (1956). 'Multiple skeletal lesions in young children due to trauma.' *J. Pediat.* **49**, 7–15

Barabas, A. P. (1967). 'Battered baby or Ehlers-Danlos syndrome?' *Lancet* **I**, 511

Barbero, G. J. and Shaheen, E. (1967). 'Environmental failure to thrive: a clinical view.' *J. Pediat.* **71**, 639–644

Barmeyer, G. H., Alderson, L. R. and Cox, W. B. (1951). 'Traumatic periostitis in young children.' *J. Pediat.* **38**, 184–190

Baron, M. A., Bejar, R. L. and Sheaff, P. J. (1970). 'Neurologic manifestations of the battered child syndrome.' *Pediatrics* **45**, 1003–1007

Benét, W. R. (1965). *The Reader's Encyclopaedia.* London: Adam and Charles Black

Bennie, E. H. and Sclare, A. B. (1969). 'The battered child syndrome.' *Am. J. Psychiat.* **125**, 975–979

Bevan, H. (1975). Should reporting be mandatory. In *Concerning Child Abuse,* Ed. by A. White Franklin. London: Churchill–Livingstone.

Birrell, R. G. and Birrell, J. H. W. (1968). The maltreatment syndrome in children: A hospital survey.' *Med. J. Aust.* **II**, 1023–1029

Bleiberg, N. (1965). 'The neglected child and the child health conference.' *N. Y. St. J. Med.* **65**, 1880–1885

Blue, M. J. (1965). 'The battered child syndrome from a social worker's viewpoint.' *Can. J. publ. Hlth* **56**, 197–198

Bluglass, R. S. (1974). Personal communication.

Boardman, H. (1962). 'A project to rescue children from inflicted injuries.' *Social Work* **7**, 43–51

Bongiovi, J. J. and Logosso, R. D. (1969). Pancreatic pseudocyst occurring in the battered child syndrome.' *J. Pediat. Surg.* **4**, 220–226

Brim, C. J. (1936). 'Medicine in the Bible.' *The Pentateuch, Torah.* New York: Froben Press

British Paediatric Association (1966). 'Memorandum by the special standing committee on accidents in childhood: The battered baby.' *Br. med. J.* **I**, 601–604

Bronson, B. H. (1959). *The Traditional Tunes of the Child Ballads,* Vol. 1. Princetown, New Jersey: Princetown University Press

Bruch, H. (1966). 'Anorexia nervosa and its differential diagnosis.' *J. nerv. ment. Dis.* **141**, 555–566.

Bryant, H. D. (1963). 'Physical abuse of children: An agency study.' *Child Welfare* **42**, 125–130

Bullard, D. M., Glaser, H. H., Heagarty, M. C. and Pivchik, E. C. (1967). 'Failure to thrive in the "neglected child". *Am. J. Orthopsych.* **37**, 680–690

Burgess, E. W. and Wallin, P. (1953). *Engagement and Marriage.* New York: Lippincott

Butler, N. R. and Alberman, E. D. (1969). 'Perinatal Problems.' *The Second Report of the 1958 British Perinatal Mortality Survey* Edinburgh and London: Livingstone

Bwibo, N. O. (1971). 'Battered child syndrome.' *E. Afr. med. J.* **48**, 56–61

Caffey, J. (1939). 'Syphilis of the skeleton in early infancy: The non-specificity of many of the roentgenographic changes.' *Am, J. Roentgen. Rad. Ther.* **42**, 637–655

Caffey, J. and Silverman, W. A. (1945). 'Infantile cortical hyperostosis: Preliminary report on a new syndrome.' *Am. J. Roentgen. rad. Ther.* **54**, 1–16

Caffey, J. (1946*a*). 'Multiple fractures in the long bones of infants suffering from chronic subdural hematoma.' *Am. J. Roentgen. rad. Ther.* **56**, 163–173

Caffey, J. (1946*b*). 'Infantile cortical hyperostoses.' *J. Pediat.* **29**, 541–549

Caffey, J. (1957). 'Some traumatic lesions in growing bones other than fractures and dislocations: Clinical and radiological features.' *Br. J. radiol.* **30**, 225–238

Caffey, J. (1965). 'Significance of the history in the diagnosis of traumatic injury to children.' *J. Pediat.* **67** (Suppl), 1008–1014

Caffey, J. (1972). 'The parent–infant traumatic stress syndrome. (Caffey-Kempe syndrome. The battered baby syndrome.)' *Am. J. Roentgen. rad. Ther. nucl. Med.* **114**, 218–229.

Caine, T. M., Foulds, G. A. and Hope, K. (1967). *Manual of the Hostility and Direction of Hostility Questionnaire.* London: University of London Press

Calef, V. (1972). 'The hostility of parents of children: Some notes on infertility, child abuse and abortion.' *Int. J. psychoanal. Psychother.* **I**, 79–96

Callaghan, K. A. and Fotheringham, B. J. (1970). 'Practical management of the battered baby syndrome.' *Med. J. Aust.* **I**, 1282–1284

Cameron, J. M. (1970). 'The battered baby.' *Br. J. hosp. Med.* **4**, 769–777

Cameron, J. M. (1972). 'The battered baby syndrome.' *Practitioner* **209**, 302–310

Cameron, J. M., Johnson, H. R. M. and Camps, F. E. (1966). 'The battered child syndrome.' *Med. Sci. & Law* **6**, 2–21

Camps, F. E. (1969). 'Injuries sustained by children from violence.' In *Recent Advances in Forensic Pathology*, Ed. by F. E. Camps. London: Churchill

Caulfield, E. (1931). *The Infant Welfare Movement in the Eighteenth Century.* New York: Hoeber

Cavenagh, W. E. (1967). *Juvenile Courts, the Child and the Law.* Harmondsworth, Middlesex: Penguin Books

Cavenagh, W. E. (1974). 'Battered baby cases in the courts.' *Justice of the Peace* **138**, 30–33

Central Health Services Council (1970). *The Battered Baby.* A memorandum prepared by the standing medical advisory committee. London: H.M.S.O.

Cheney, K. B. (1966). 'Safeguarding legal rights in providing protective services.' *Children* **13**, 86–92

Cherry, B. J. and Kuby, A. M. (1971). 'Obstacles to the delivery of medical care to children of neglecting parents.' *Am. J. publ. Hlth* **61**, 568–573

Chesser, E. (1952). *Cruelty to Children.* New York: Philosophical Library

Chichester Psychiatric Service (1962). 'Home visit schedule.' In *The Burden on the Community. The Epidemiology of Mental Illness: A symposium.* Nuffield Provincial Hospitals Trust. London: Oxford University Press

Children and Young Persons Act 1963. Part I, Section 1. London: H.M.S.O.

Children's Bureau (1966). *The Child Abuse Reporting Laws: A Tabular View.* Washington D. C. Social and Rehabilitation Service. Department of Health, Education and Welfare

City of Birmingham (1972). *Abstracts of Statistics (1970–1).* Central Statistics Office: City of Birmingham

Cobb, W. A. (1963). 'The normal adult EEG.' In *Electroencephalography,* Ed. by D. Hill and G. Parr. London: Macdonald

Cochrane, W. (1965). 'The battered child syndrome.' *Can. J. publ. Hlth* **56,** 193–196

Cohen, M. I., Raphling, D. L. and Green, P. E. (1966). 'Psychologic aspects of the maltreatment syndrome of childhood.' *J. Pediat.* **69**, 279–284

Colclough, I. R. (1972). 'Victorian government's report on child abuse: A re-investigation.' *Med. J. Aust.* **II**, 1491–1497

Colman, A. D. and Colman, L. L. (1971). *Pregnancy: The Psychological Experience.* New York: Herder and Herder

Cooper, C. E. (1970). 'Battered babies.' *J. med. Wom. Fed.* **52**, 93–98

Cooper, C. E. (1974). Personal communication.

Corbett, J. T. (1964). 'A psychiatrist reviews the battered child syndrome and mandatory reporting legislation.' *NW Med.* **63**, 920–922

Court, J. (1969). 'The battered child: Historical and diagnostic reflections on treatment.' *Med. Social Work* **22**, 11–20

Court, J. (1973)., 'Some reflections on non-accidental injury to young children.' *Social Work Service,* No. 3, 6–10. Issued by Social Work Service Department, D.H.S.S.

Court, J. and Kerr, A. (1971). ' The battered child syndrome. 2. A preventable disease?' *Nursing Times* **67**, 695–697

Craft, M. (1969). 'The natural history of psychopathic disorder.' *Br. J. Psychiat.* **115,** 39–44

Crellin, E., Pringle, M. L., Kellmer and West, P. (1971). *Born Illegitimate, Social and Educational Implications.* London: National Foundation for Educational Research in England and Wales

Crisp, A. H. (1967). 'Anorexia nervosa.' *Hosp. Med.* **1**, 713–718

Crisp, A. H. (1971). Personal communication

Cronbach, L. (1960). *Essentials of Psychological Testing.* Harper and Row.

Cross, K. W. (1973). Personal communication

Crosse, V. M. (1971). *The Pre-term Baby and other Babies with Low Birth Weight.* Edinburgh and London: Churchill, Livingstone

Curtis, G. (1973). 'Violence breeds violence – perhaps?' *Am. J. Psychiat.* **120,** 386–387

Darwin, C. (1936). *The Origin of Species and the Descent of Man.* New York: Modern Library

Davids, A. and Holden, R. H. (1970). 'Consistency of maternal attitudes and personality from pregnancy to eight months following childbirth.' *Dev. Psychol.* **2**, 364–366

Davis, K. (1973). 'The theory of change and response in modern demographic history.' *Popul. Index* **29**, 345–366

Davoren, E. (1968). 'The role of the social worker.' In *The Battered Child,* Ed. by R. E. Helfer and C. H. Kempe. Chicago: University of Chicago Press

De Francis, V. (1963). *Child Abuse: Preview of a Nationwide Survey.* Denver, Colorado, Children's Division, American Humane Association

De Francis, V. (1972). 'The status of child protective services. A national dilemma.' In *Helping the Battered Child and His Family,* Ed. by C. H. Kempe and R. E. Helfer. Philadelphia and Toronto: J. B. Lippincott

De Lissovoy, V. (1973). 'High school marriages: A longitudinal study.' *J. marriage Fam.* **35**, 245–255

Delsordo, J. (1963). 'Protective casework for abused children.' *Children* **10**, 213–218

Department of Health and Social Security (1972). The battered baby syndrome. An analysis of reports submitted by medical officers of health and children's officers. London: H.M.S.O.

Department of Health and Social Security Library (1973). Selected references on child abuse. 1968–1973. London: D.H.S.S.

Department of Health and Social Security (1974). Non-accidental injury to children. London: D.H.S.S.

Department of Health and Social Security (1974). Report of the Committee of Inquiry into the Care and Supervision Provided in Relation to Maria Colwell. London: H.M.S.O.

Diggle, G. and Jackson, G. (1973). 'Child injury intensive monitoring system.' *Br. med. J.* **III**, 334–335

Dine, M. S. (1965). 'Tranquillizer poisoning. An example of child abuse.' *Pediatrics* **36**, 782–785

Doll, E. A. (1947). *Vineland Social Maturity Scale. Manual of Directions.* Minneapolis, Minnesota Educational Test Bureau

D'Orban, P. (1974). Personal communication

Drillien, C. M. (1964). *The Growth and Development of the Prematurely Born Infant.* Edinburgh and London: Livingstone

Dunn, C. (1920). *The Natural History of the Child.* New York: John Lane

Easson, W. M. and Steinhilber, R. M. (1961). 'Murderous aggression by children and adolescents.' *Archs gen. Psychiat.* **4**, 1–10

Ebbin, A. J., Gollub, M. H., Stein, A. M. and Wilson, M. G. (1969). 'Battered child syndrome at the Los Angeles County General Hospital.' *Am. J. Dis. Child.* **118**, 660–667

Eddy, W. A. (1965). *Satires and Personal Writings,* Ed. by W. A. Eddy. London: Oxford University Press

Eisenstein, E. M., Delta, B. G. and Clifford, J. H. (1965). 'Jejunal hematoma: An unusual manifestation of the battered child syndrome.' *Clin. Pediat.* **4**, 436–440

Elmer, E. (1960). 'Abused young children seen in hospitals.' *Social Work* **5**, 98–102

Elmer, E. (1963). 'Identification of abused children.' *Children* **10**, 180–184

Elmer, E. (1967). *Children in Jeopardy: A Study of Abused Minors and their Families.* Pittsburgh: University of Pittsburgh Press

Elmer, E. and Gregg, G. S. (1967). 'Developmental characteristics of abused children.' *Pediatrics* **4**, 596–602

Emery, J. L. (1972). 'Welfare of families of children found unexpectedly dead ("cot deaths").' *Br. med. J.* **I**, 612–615

Encyclopaedia Britannica (1890). 9th Edition. Vol. 13. Edinburgh: A. and C. Black

Eysenck, H. J. (1964). *Crime and Personality.* London: Routledge and Kegan Paul

Eysenck, H. J. and Eysenck, S. B. G. (1964). *Manual of the Eysenck Personality Inventory.* London: University of London Press

Fairburn, A. C. and Hunt, A. C. (1964). 'Caffey's "third syndrome" : A critical evaluation ("The battered baby").' *Med. Sc. & Law* **4**, 123–126

Farrington, D. P. and West, D. J. (1971). 'A comparison between early delinquents and young aggressives.' *Br. J. Criminol.* **11**, 341–358

Feinstein, H. M., Paul, N. and Esmiol, P. (1964). 'Group therapy for mothers with infanticidal impulses.' *Am. J. Psychiat.* **120**, 882–886

Fetherstone, W. M. (1972). 'Nobody's baby?' *Law Soc. Gaz.* **69**, 873

Fiser, R. H., Kaplan, J. and Holder , J. C. (1972). 'Congenital syphilis mimicking the battered child syndrome: How does one tell them apart?' *Clin. Pediat.* **11**, 305–307

Fisher, S. H. (1958). 'Skeletal manifestations of parent induced trauma in infants and children.' *Sth. med. J.* **51**, 956–960

Fleming, G. M. (1967). 'Cruelty to children.' *Br. med. J.* **II**, 421–422

Fontana, V. J., Donovan, D. and Wong, R. J. (1963). 'The maltreatment syndrome in children.' *New Engl. J. Med.* 269, 1389–1394

Fontana, V. J. (1964). 'The neglect and abuse of children.' *N. Y. St. J. Med.* 64, 215–224

Fontana, V. J. (1966). 'Recognition and prevention of the battered child syndrome.' *Pediatrics* **38**, 1078

Fontana, V. J. (1968). 'Further reflections on maltreatment of children.' *N. Y. St. J. Med* **68**, 2214–2215

Fontana, V. J. (1970). ' Physical abuse of children.' *Pediatrics* **45**, 509–510

Fontana, V. J. (1971). *The Maltreated Child. The Maltreatment Syndrome in Children.* Springfield, Illinois: Charles C. Thomas

Freud, S. (1950). *Collected Papers,* Volume 2. London: Hogarth

Friedman, M. S. (1958). 'Traumatic periostitis in infants and children.' *J. Am. med. Ass.* **166**, 1840–1845

Friedman, S. B. (1970). Personal communication

Galdston, R. (1965). 'Observations on children who have been physically abused and their parents.' *Am. J. Psychiat.* **122**, 440–443

Galdston, R. (1966). *Proceedings of Conference on Patterns of Parental Behaviour Leading to Physical Abuse of Children.* University of Colorado School of Medicine. Unpublished

Galdston, R. (1971). 'Violence begins at home. The parents center project for the study and prevention of child abuse.' *J. Am. Acad. child Psychiat.* **10**, 336–350

Garner, H. (1967). 'Confrontation techniques may help "child battering" parent.' *Roche Rep.* (*Frontiers hosp. Psychiat.*) **4**, 1–11

Garrison, F. H. (1965). *Abt-Garrison History of Pediatrics,* Reprinted from *Pediatrics* by various authors. Volume 1 Ed. by J. A. Abt. Philadelphia and London: W. B. Saunders

Gibbens, T. C. N. and Walker. A. (1956). *Cruel Parents.* London: Institute for the Study and Treatment of Delinquency

Gibbs, F. A. and Gibbs, E. L. (1952). *Atlas of Electroencephalography* Cambridge, Massachusetts: Addison – Wesley

Gibson, A. G. (1973). 'Non-accidental injury to children.' *Br. med. J.* **IV**, 359

Gibson, H. B. (1964). 'The Spiral Maze. A psychomotor test with implications for the study of delinquency.' *Br. J. Psychol.* **55**, 219–225

Gibson, H. B. (1965). *Manual of the Gibson Spiral Maze.* London: University of London Press

Gibson, H. B. (1969). 'Early delinquency in relation to broken homes.' *J. child Psychol. Psychiat.* **10**, 195–204

Gil, D. G. (1968*a*). 'California pilot study.' In *The Battered Child,* Ed. by R. E. Helfer and C. H. Kempe. Chicago: University of Chicago Press

Gil, D. G. (1968*b*). 'Incidence of child abuse and demographic characteristics of persons involved.' In *The Battered Child,* Ed. by R. E. Helfer and C. H. Kempe. Chicago: University of Chicago Press

Gil, D. G. (1969). 'Physical abuse of children: Findings and implications of a nationwide survey.' *Pediatrics* (Suppl.) **44**, 857–864

Gil, D. G. (1970). *Violence Against Children. Physical Abuse in the United States.* Cambridge, Massachusetts: Harvard University Press

Gilkes, M. J. and Mann, T.P. (1967). 'Fundi of battered babies.' *Lancet* **II**, 468–469

Gillespie, R. W. (1965). 'The battered child syndrome: Thermal and caustic manifestations.' *J. Trauma* **5**, 523–525

Gluckman, L. K. (1968). 'Cruelty to children.' *N.Z. med. J.* **67**, 155–159

Glueck, S. and Glueck, E. (1962). *Delinquents and Non-Delinquents in Perspective.* Cambridge, Massachusetts: Harvard University Press

Godfrey, E. (1907). *English Children in Olden Times.* London: Methuen

Goldberg, D. P. (1972). *The Detection of Psychiatric Illness by Questionnaire. A Technique for the Identification and Assessment of Non-Psychotic Psychiatric Illness.* London: Oxford University Press

Goode, W. J. (1966). 'A sociological perspective on marital dissolution.' In *Sociology of the Family,* Ed. by M. Anderson. Harmondsworth, Middlesex: Penguin Books (1971).

Goodman, L. and Power, M. (1973). Children under 17 years of age resident in inner London subject to care proceedings, July 1971–June, 1972. A paper presented at the study group on non-accidental injury to children, Tunbridge Wells, Kent. Unpublished

Goodman, K. L. (1974).'The children and young persons acts, 1969: A case of neglect or ill treatment.' *Justice of the Peace* **138**, 6–8

Goodman, L. (1973). Personal communication

Gorer, G. (1955). *Exploring English Character.* London: The Cresset Press

Gorer, G. (1968). 'Man has no "killer instinct".' In *Man and Aggression*, Ed. by Ashley Montagu. London: Oxford University Press

Gornall, P., Ahmed, S., Jolleys, A. and Cohen, S. J. (1972). 'Intra-abdominal injuries in the battered baby syndrome.' *Archs Dis. Child.* **47**, 211–214

Graham-Hall, J. (1975). In *Concerning Child Abuse,* Ed. by A. White Franklin. London: Churchill-Livingstone

Green, K. (1965). 'Diagnosing the battered child syndrome.' *Md St. med. J.* **14**, 83–84

Greengard, J. (1964). 'The battered child syndrome.' *Am. J. Nurs.* **64**, 98–100

Greenland, C. (1973). *Child Abuse in Ontario. Research Report 3.* Ontario Ministry of Community and Social Services Research and Planning Branch.

Gregg, G. S. (1968). 'Physicians, child abuse, reporting laws, and injured child: Psychosocial anatomy of childhood trauma. *Clin. Pediat.* **7**, 720–725

Gregg, G. S. and Elmer, E. (1969). 'Infant injuries: Accident or abuse?' *Pediatrics* **44**, 443–449

Griffiths, D. L. and Moynihan, F. J. (1963). 'Multiple epiphyseal injuries in babies ("battered baby" syndrome).' *Br. med. J.* **II**, 1558–1561

Griffiths, M. I. (1974). Personal communication

Griffiths, R. (1954). *The Abilities of Babies. A Study in Mental Measurement.* London: University of London Press

Griffiths, R. (1967). *Record Book for Use with the Griffiths Mental Developmental Scales for Testing Babies and Young Children From Birth to Eight Years of Age.* Taunton: Development Research Centre

Guthkelch, A. N. (1971). 'Infantile subdural haematoma and its relationship to whiplash injuries.' *Br. med. J.* **II**, 430–431

Gwinn, J. L., Lewin, K. W. and Peterson, H. G., Jr. (1961). 'Roentgenographic manifestations of unsuspected trauma in infancy: A problem of medical, social and legal importance.' *J. Am. med. Ass.* **176**, 926–929

Hall, M. H. (1975). 'A view from the emergency and accident department.' In *Concerning Child Abuse*, Ed. by A. White Franklin., London: Churchill-Livingstone

Hall, M. H. (1974). Personal communication

Hamlin, H. (1968). 'Subgaleal hematoma caused by hair-pull. *J. Am. med. Ass.* **204**, 339

Harcourt, B. and Hopkins, D. (1971). 'Ophthalmic manifestations of the battered baby syndrome.' *Br. med. J.* **III**, 398–401

Harding, G. (1973). Personal communication.

Hare, R. D. (1972). 'Depression.' In *Encyclopaedia of Psychology*, Ed. by H. J. Eysenck, W. A. Arnold and R. Meili, London: Research Press

Harper, F. V. (1963). 'The physician, the battered child and the law.' *Pediatrics* **31**, 899–902

Hartley, S. F. (1971). 'Contributions of illegitimate and pre-maritally conceived births to total fertility.' *Soc. Biol.* **18**, 178–187

Heins, M. (1969). 'Child abuse: Analysis of a current epidemic.' *Mich. Med.* **68**, 887–891

Heise, D. R. (1970). 'The semantic differential and attitude research.' In *Attitude Measurement*, Ed. by G. F. Summers. Chicago: Rand McNally

Helfer, R. E. (1968). 'The responsibility and role of the physician.' In *The Battered Child*, Ed. by R. E. Helfer and C. H. Kempe. Chicago: University of Chicago Press

Helfer, R. E. (1970). 'Physical abuse of children.' *Pediatrics* **45**, 651–652

Helfer, R. E. (1973). 'Foreword to The Battered Child in Canada. (Van Stolk, 1972). op. cit.

Helfer, R. E. and Kempe, C. H. (1968). *The Battered Child*, Ed. by R. E. Helfer and C. H. Kempe. Chicago: University of Chicago Press

Helfer, R. E. and Pollock, C. H. (1968). 'The battered child syndrome.' *Adv. Pediat.* **15**, 9–27

Heywood, J. S. (1965). *Children in Care. The Development of the Service for the Deprived Child.* London: Routledge and Kegan Paul

Hill, D. (1943). 'Cerebral dysrhythmia: Its significance in aggressive behaviour.' *Proc. R. Soc. Med.* **37**, 317–328

Hill, D. and Watterson, D. (1942). 'Electro-encephalographic studies of psychopathic personalities.' *J. Neurol. Psychiat.* **5**, 47–65

Hiller, R. B. (1969). 'The battered child. A health visitor's point of view.' *Nursing Times* **65**, 1265–1266

Hindley, C. B. (1960). The Griffiths scale of infant development: Scores and predictions from 3 to 18 months. *J. child Psychol. Psychiat.* **1**, 99–112

Hindley, C. B. (1965). 'Stability and change in abilities up to five years: Group trends.' *J. child Psychol. Psychiat.* **6**, 85–99

Hobhouse, N. (1938). Comment on 'pre-psychotic anorexia' (paper by G. Nicolle). *Lancet*, **ii**, 1174

Holter, J. C. and Friedman, S. B. (1968*a*). 'Child abuse: Early case finding in the emergency department.' *Pediatrics* **42**, 128–138

Holter, J. C. and Friedman, S. B. (1968*b*) 'Principles of management in child abuse cases.' *Am. J. Orthopsychiat.* **38**, 127–136

Honzik, M. P. (1957). 'Developmental studies of parent–child resemblance in intelligence.' *Child Dev.* **28**, 215–228

Horobin, G. (Editor) (1973). *Experience with Abortion: A Case Study of North East England.* London: Cambridge University Press

Howells, J. G. (1974). *Remember Maria.* London: Butterworth

Ingraham, F. D. and Heyl, H. L. (1939). 'Subdural hematoma in infancy and childhood.' *J. Am. med. Ass.* **122,** 198–204

Ingram, H. W. F. (1973). *A Note on Reporting.* A paper presented at the study group on non-accidental injury to children at Tunbridge Wells, Kent. Unpublished.

Isaacs, S. (1968). 'Physical ill-treatment of children. *Lancet* **I,** 37

Isaacs, S. (1972). 'Neglect, cruelty and battering.' *Br. med. J.* **III,** 224–226

Jackson, G. (1972). 'Child abuse syndrome: The cases we miss.' *Br. med. J.* **II,** 756–757

Jacobziner, H. (1964). 'Rescuing the battered child.' *Am. J. Nurs.* **64,** 92–97

Jeavons, P. M. and Bower, B. D. (1974). 'Infantile spasms.' In *Handbook of Clinical Neurology,* Ed. by P. J. Vinken and G. W. Bruyn. Amsterdam: North Holland

Jenkins, R. L. (1954). 'The significance of maternal rejection of pregnancy for the future development of the child.' In *Therapeutic Abortion. Medical, Psychiatric, Legal and Anthropological and Religious Considerations,* Ed. by H. Rosen. New York: The Julian Press

Johnson, B. and Morse, H. A. (1968). 'Injured children and their parents.' *Children* **15,** 147–152

Joos, T. H. (1969). 'Child abuse: A different point of view.' *Pediatrics* **45,** 511

J. Am med. Ass. (1962). Editorial. 'The battered child syndrome.' **181**, 42

J. Am. med. Ass. (1964). Editorial. 'Battered child legislation.' **181**, 386

Kaufman, I. (1962). 'Psychiatric implications of physical abuse of children.' In *Protecting the Battered Child,* Ed. by V. de Francis. Denver, Colorado: American Humane Association

Kempe, C. H. (1968). 'Some problems encountered by welfare departments in the management of the battered child syndrome.' In *The Battered Child,* Ed. by R. E. Helfer and C. H. Kempe. Chicago: University of Chicago Press.

Kempe, C. H. (1969). 'The battered child and the hospital.' *Hosp. Pract.* **4,** 44–57

Kempe, C. H. (1970). Quoted in Cameron, J. M. (1970). 'The battered baby syndrome.' *Br. J. hosp. Med.* **4,** 769–777

Kempe, C. H. (1971). 'Pediatric implications of the battered baby syndrome.' *Archs Dis. Childh.* **46,** 28–37

Kempe, C. H. (1973). Position paper for hearings of the subcommittee on children and youth of the committee on labour and public welfare. United States Senate, March 31, 1973, Denver, Colorado. Unpublished

Kempe, C. H. and Helfer, R. E. (1972). *Helping the Battered Child and his Family,* Ed. by C. H. Kempe and R. E. Helfer. Philadelphia and Toronto: J. B. Lippincott

Kempe, C. H. and Helfer, R. E. (1972). 'Innovative therapeutic approaches.' In *Helping the Battered Child and His Family,* Ed. by C. H. Kempe and R. E. Helfer. Philadelphia and Toronto: J. B. Lippincott

Kempe, C. H., Silverman, F. N., Steele, B. F., Droegemueller, W. and Silver, H. K. (1962). 'The battered child syndrome.' *J. Am. med. Ass.* **181,** 17–24

Kiffney, G. T., Jr. (1964). 'The eye of the battered child.' *Archs Ophthal.* **72,** 231–233

Klaus, M. H. and Kennell, J. H. (1970). 'Mothers separated from their newborn infants.' *Pediat. Clins. N. Am.* **17,** 1015–1037

Klein, M. and Stern, L. (1971). 'Low birth weight and the battered child syndrome.' *Am. J. Dis. Child.* **122**, 15–18

Koel, B. S., (1969). ' Failure to thrive and fatal injury as a continuum.' *Am. J. Dis. Child.* **118**, 565–567

Komisaruk, R. (1966). 'Clinical evaluation of child abuse: Scarred families, a preliminary report.' *Juv. Court Judg. J. (Wayne Co., Mich.)* **17**, 66–70

Korsch, B. M., Christian, J. B., Gozzi, E. K. and Carolson, P. V. (1965). 'Infant care and punishment. A pilot study.' *Am. J. Publ. Hlth* **55**, 1880–1888

Köttgen, U. (1967). 'Kindesmisshandlung.' *Mschr. Kinderheilk.* **115**, 186–192

Kramer, S. N. (1956). *From the Tablets of Sumer: Twenty-five Firsts in Man's Recorded History.* Indian Hills, Colorado: Falcon's Wing

Kreitman, N., Joyce, C., Barbara, N. and Jane, J. (1970). 'Neurosis and marital interaction – II.' *Br. J. Psychiat.* **117**, 47–58

Krige, H. N. (1966). 'The abused child complex and its characteristic x-ray findings.' *S. Afr. med. J.* **40**, 490–493

Kroeger, N. (1965). A survey of physically abused children known to selected hospitals and health agencies in the Chicago area, 1964. Publication No. 4008. Chicago. Welfare Council of Metropolitan Chicago

Kunstadter, R. H., Singer, M. H. and Steinberg, R. (1967). 'The "battered child" and the celiac syndrome.' *Ill. med. J.* **132**, 267–272

Lancet, (1971). Editorial. Violent parents. **2**, 1017–1018

Laupus, W. E., (1966). 'Child abuse and the physician.' The *Va med. Mon.* **93**, 1–2

Leonard, M. F., Rhymes, J. P. and Solnit, A. J. (1966). 'Failure to thrive in infants: A family problem.' *Am. J. Dis. Child.* **111**, 600–612

Levy, P. (1968). 'Short-form tests. A methodological review. *Psychol. Bull.* **69**, 410–416

Lis, E. F. and Frauenberger, G. S. (1950). 'Multiple fractures associated with subdural hematoma in infancy.' *Pediatrics* **6**, 890–892

Low, C. (1971). 'The battering parent, the community and the law.' *Appl. Soc. Stud.* **3**, 65–80

Luke, J. L., Lyons, M. M. and Devlin, J. F. (1967). 'Pediatric forensic pathology. I. Death by homicide.' *J. forens. Sci.* **12**, 421–430

Lukianowicz, N. (1969). 'Parental maltreatment of children.' *Br. J. soc. Psychiat.* **3**, 189–195

Lukianowicz, N. (1971). 'Battered children.' *Psychiat. Clin.* **4**, 257–280

Macdonald, J. (1963). 'The threat to kill.' *Am. J. Psychiat.* **120**, 125–130

Mackeith, R. (1974). 'Speculations on non-accidental injury as a cause of chronic brain disorder.' *Dev. Med. Child Neurol.* **16**, 216–218

Makover, H. (1966). Proceedings of conference on patterns of parental behaviour leading to physical abuse of children. University of Colorado School of Medicine. Unpublished

Malinowski, B. (1927). *Sex and Repression in Savage Society.* New York: Harcourt, Brace and World

Malone, C. A. (1966). 'Safety first' Comments on the influence of external danger in the lives of children of disorganized families.' *Am. J. Orthopsychiat.* **36**, 3–12

Manson, G. (1964). 'Neglected children and the celiac syndrome.' *J. Iowa med. Soc.* **54**, 228–234

Maroteaux, P. and Fessard, C. (1969). 'La maladie des enfants battus – syndrome de Silverman.' *Concours méd.* **91**, 6704–6711

Maroteaux, P. and Lamy, M. (1967). 'Fundi of battered babies.' *Lancet* **II**, 829

Marquézy, R. A., Bach, Ch. and Blondeau, M. (1952). 'Hématome sous-dural fractures multiples des os longs chez unnourrisson de 9 mois.' *Archs fr. Pédiat.*, 526–531

Martin, H. (1972). 'The child and his development.' In *Helping the Battered Child and His Family.* Ed. by C. H. Kempe and R. E. Helfer. Oxford: J. B. Lippincott

Maxwell, E. (1957). 'Validities of abbreviated W.A.I.S. scales.' *J. Consult. Psychol.* **21**, 121–126

Maxwell, I. D. (1966). 'Assault and battery of children and others.' *Nova Scotia med. Bull.* **45**, 105–107

Mayer-Gross, W., Slater, E. and Roth, M. (1969). *Clinical Psychiatry.* Third Edition. London,Bailliere, Tindall and Cassell

Mayo, P. R. (1966). 'Speed and accuracy of depression on a Spiral Maze Test.' *Percept. Motor Skills* **23**, 1034

McCoid, A. H. (1965). 'The battered child and other assaults upon the family – I.' *Minn. Law Rev.* **50**, 1–50

McCord, W., McCord, J. and Zola, I. K. (1959). *Origins of Crime.* New York: Columbia University Press

McCort, J. and Vaudagna, J. (1964). 'Visceral injuries in battered children.' *Radiology* **82**, 424–428

McFerran, J. (1958). 'Parent groups in protective services.' *Children* **5**, 223–228

McHenry, T., Girdany, B. R. and Elmer, E. (1963). 'Unsuspected trauma with multiple skeletal injuries during infancy and childhood.' *Pediatrics* **31**, 903–908

Mead, M. (1928). *Coming of Age in Samoa.* New York: Morrow

Medical Defence Union (1966). Battered babies. In *Annual Report,* pp. 18–20

Megargee, E. I. (1966). 'Undercontrolled and overcontrolled personality types in extreme antisocial aggression'. *Psychol. Monogr. Gen. Appl.* **80**, No. 611

Melnick, R. and Hurley, J. R. (1969). 'Distinctive personality attributes of child abusing mothers.' *J. consult. clin. Psychol.* **33**, 746–749

Menninger, K. (1942). *Love Against Hate.* New York: Harcourt, Brace

Merrill, E. J. (1962). 'Physical abuse of children: An agency study.' In *Protecting the Battered Child,* Ed. by V. de Francis. Denver, Colorado: Children's Division, American Humane Association

Miller, D. S. (1959). 'Fractures among children – I. Parental assault as causative agent.' *Minn. Med.* **42**, 1209–1213

Millichap, J. G., Bickford, R. G., Klaus, D. W. and Backus, R. E. (1962). 'Infantile spasms, hypoarhythmia and mental retardation. A study of etiological factors in 61 patients.'

Milowe, I. D. (1966). Proceedings of conference on patterns of parental behaviour leading to physical abuse of children. University of Colorado School of Medicine. Unpublished

Milowe, I. D. and Lourie, R. S. (1964). ' The child's role in the battered child syndrome.' *J. Pediat.* **65**, 1079–1081

Monckton, W. (1945). Report on the circumstances which led to the boarding-out of Dennis and Terence O'Neill at Bank Farm, Ministerly and the steps taken to supervise their welfare. London: H.M.S.O.

Morris, M. G. and Gould, R. W. (1963). 'Role reversal: A necessary concept in dealing with the "battered child syndrome".' *Am. J. Orthopsychiat.* **33**, 298–299

Morris, M. G., Gould, R. W. and Matthews, P. J. (1964). 'Toward prevention of child abuse.' *Children* **11**, 55–60

Morse, C. W., Sahler, O. J. Z. and Friedman, S. B. (1970). 'A three-year follow-up study of abused and neglected children.' *Am. J. Dis. Child.* **120**, 439–446

Mounsey, J. (1974). Personal communication

Mounsey, J. (1975). 'Offences of criminal violence, cruelty and neglect against children in Lancashire.' In *Concerning Child Abuse,* Ed. by A. White Franklin. London: Churchill-Livingstone.

Mushin, A. S. (1971). 'Ocular damage in the battered baby syndrome.' *Br. med. J.* **III**, 402–404

Nathan, H. (1965). 'Abused children.' *Am. J. Psychiat.* **122**, 443

National Library of Medicine (1973). Literature Search No. 72–28. Child abuse: January, 1970 through July, 1973. U. S. Department of Health, Education and Welfare. Public Health Service, National Institute of Health

Neimann, N. and Rabouille, D. (1969). 'Les enfants victimes de sévices.' *Revue Pract.* **19**, 3879–3888

Newson, J. (1973*a*). Personal communication

Newson, J. (1973*b*). 'Towards a theory of infant understanding.' Unpublished paper.

Newson, J. and Newson, E. (1963). *Patterns of Infant Care in an Urban Community.* London: Allen and Unwin (Penguin Books, 1972)

Newson, J. and Newson E. (1968). *Four Years Old in an Urban Community.* London: Allen and Unwin (Pelican Books 1970)

New Society (1973). 'Caring for children.' **24**, 542

Nie, N. N., Bent, D. H. and Hodlaihull, C. (1970). *Statistical Package for the Social Sciences.* London: McGraw-Hill

Nixon, H. H. and Court, S. D. M. (1973). 'Non-accidental injury in children: Introductory comment from B.P.A. and B.P.A.S.' *Br. med. J.* **IV**, 656–657

Nomura, F. M. (1966). 'The battered child syndrome. A review.' *Hawaii med. J.* **25**, 387–394

Non-accidental Injury in Children (1973). 'A guide on management; prepared by a working party in the department of child health, University of Newcastle Upon Tyne.' *Br. med. J.* **4**, 657–660

Nurse, S. M. (1966). 'Familial patterns of parents who abuse their children.' *Smith Coll. Stud. soc. Work* **35**, 11–25

Oettinger, K. B. (1968). Foreword to *The Battered Child,* Ed. by R. E. Helfer and C. H. Kempe. Chicago: University of Chicago Press

Okell, C. (1971). 'Childhood accidents and child abuse.' *Community Med.* **126**, 124–127

Oliver, J. E. (1974). Personal communication

Oliver, J. E. and Taylor, A. (1971). 'Five generations of ill-treated children in one family pedigree.' *Br. J. Psychiat.* **119**, 473–480

Oliver, J. E. and Cox, J. (1973). 'A family kindred with ill-used children: The burden on the community.' *Br. J. Psychiat.* **123**, 81–90

Oliver, J. E., Cox, J., Taylor, A. and Baldwin, J. A. (1974). Severely ill-treated young children in north-east Wiltshire. Research Report No. 4. Oxford Record Linkage Study. Oxford Regional Health Authority.

Opie, I. and Opie, P. (1974) *The Classic Fairy Tales.* London: Oxford University Press

Osborn, F. (1963). 'Excess and unwanted fertility.' *Eugen. Q.* **10**, 59–72

Osgood, C. E., Suci, G. J. and Tannenbaum, P. H. (1957). *The Measurement of Meaning.* Urbana, Illinois: University of Illinois Press

Ounsted, C. (1968). 'Battered baby syndrome. A review of a tape recording made by K. Simpson for the Royal College of General Practitioners.' *Dev. Med. child Neurol.* **10**, 133–134

Ounsted, C. (1972). *Proceedings of the Eighth International Study Group on Child Neurology and Cerebral Palsy.* Unpublished.

Ounsted, C., Oppenheimer, R. and Lindsay, J. (1974). 'Aspects of bonding failure: The psychopathology and psychotherapeutic treatment of families of battered children? *Dev. Med. child Neurol.* **16,** 447–456

Owen, D. (1974). Personal communication

Pashayan, H., and Cochrane, W. H. (1965). 'Maltreatment syndrome of children.' *Nova Scotia med. Bull.* **44,** 139–142

Patton, R. G. and Gardner, L. I. (1962). 'Influence of family environment on growth: The syndrome of maternal deprivation.' *Pediatrics* **30,** 957–962

Paul, S. D. (1972). 'Recognition of the entity "the battered child" syndrome in India.' *Indian J. Pediat.* **39,** 58–62

Paulsen, M. G. (1966). 'Legal protections against child abuse.' *Children* **13,** 42–48

Paulsen, M. G. (1967). 'Child abuse reporting laws: The shape of the legislation.' *Columbia Law Rev.* **67,** 1–49.

Paulsen, M. G. (1968). 'The law and abused children.' In *The Battered Child,* Ed. by R. E. Helfer and C. H. Kempe. Chicago: University of Chicago Press.

Paulson, M. J. and Blake, P. R. (1967). 'The abused, battered and maltreated child. A review.' *Trauma* **9,** 3–136

Paulsen, M. G., Parker, G. and Adelman, L. (1966). 'Child abuse reporting law: Some legislative history.' *George Washington Law Rev.* **34,** 482–506

Paulson, M. J. and Blake, P. R. (1969). 'The physically abused child. A focus on prevention.' *Child Welf.* **48,** 86–95

Paulson, M. J., Savino, A. B., Chaleff, A. B. and Wyman Sanders, R. (1971). Group psychotherapy: A multidisciplinary approach in the treatment of abusive parents. Unpublished

Phaire, T. (1545). *The Boke of Chyldren.* Edinburgh and London: E and S Livingstone (1955)

Phelps, C. D. (1971). 'The association of pale centred retinal hemorrhages with intracranial bleeding in infancy.' *Am. J. Ophthal.* **72,** 348–350

Philip, A. E. (1969). 'The development and use of hostility and direction of hostility questionnaire.' *J. psychosom. Res.* **13,** 283–287

Phillips, C. J., Wilson, H. and Herbert, G. W. (1972). Child Development Study (Birmingham 1968–71): A Study of Inadequate Families. Part 1. A Report to the Department of Health and Social Security and the Bernard van Leer Foundation. Centre for Child Study, School of Education, University of Birmingham

Pickel, S., Anderson, C. and Holliday (1970). 'Thirsting and hypernatremic dehydration: A form of child abuse.' *Pediatrics* **45,** 54–59

Platou, R. V., Lennox, R. and Beasley, J. D. (1964). 'Battering.' *Bull. Tulane med. Fac.* **23,** 157–165

Pohlman, E. (1973). *The Psychology of Birth Planning.* Cambridge Massachusetts: Schenkman

Polansky, N. (1968). The current status on child abuse and child neglect in this country. Report to the Joint Commission on Mental Health for Children (Quoted in Gil, D. G. 1970. Violence Against Children. Physical Abuse in the United States. Cambridge, Massachusetts: Harvard University Press)

Pollak, M. (1972). *Todays Three Year Olds in London.* London: William Heinemann

Potter, C. F. (1949). 'Infanticides.' In *Dictionary of Folklore, Mythology and Legend,* Ed. by M. Leach, Vol. 1. New York: Funk and Wagnalls

Pringle, M. L. K. (1969). *Social Learning and its Measurement.* London: Longmans, Green and Co.

Radbill, S. X. (1968). 'A history of child abuse and infanticide.' In *The Battered Child,* Ed. by R. E. Helfer and C. H. Kempe. Chicago: University of Chicago Press

Registrar General (1969). *Statistical Review of England and Wales for the year 1967.* Part 3. London: H.M.S.O.

Registrar General (1970). *Statistical Review of England and Wales for the year 1968.* Part 3. London: H.M.S.O.

Registrar General (1971). *Statistical Review of England and Wales for the year 1969.* Part 3. London: H.M.S.O.

Registrar General (1972*a*). *Statistical Review of England and Wales for 1970.* Part 2. London: H.M.S.O.

Registrar General (1972*b*). *Statistical Review of England and Wales for the year 1970.* Part 3. London: H.M.S.O.

Registrar General (1973). *Statistical Review of England and Wales for the year 1971.* Part 2. London: H.M.S.O.

Reiner, B. S. and Kaufman, I. (1959). *Character Disorders in Parents of Delinquents.* New York: Family Service Association of America

Resnick, P. J. (1969). 'Murder of the newborn: A psychiatric review of neonaticide.' *Am. J. Psychiat.* **126**, 1414–1420

Resnick, P. J. (1972). 'Infanticide.' In *Modern Perspectives in Psycho-Obstetrics,* Ed. by J. G. Howells. Edinburgh: Oliver and Boyd

Richards, I. D. G. and McIntosh, H. T. (1972). 'Confidential inquiry into 226 consecutive infant deaths.' *Archs Dis. Childh.* **47**, 697–706

Robins, L. N. (1966). *Deviant Children Grown Up. A Sociological and Psychiatric Study of Sociopathic Personality.* Baltimore: Williams and Wilkins

Robinson, H. (1973). Personal communication

Rose, C. B. (1936). 'Unusual periostitis in children.' *Radiology* **27**, 131–137

Ross, T. A. (1938). 'Comment on "pre-psychotic anorexia" (paper by G. Nicolle).' *Lancet,* **ii**, 1173

Rowntree, G. (1964). 'Some aspects of marriage breakdown in Britain during the last 30 years.' *Popul. Stud.* **18**, 147–163

Royston Pike, R. (1966). *Human Documents of the Industrial Revolution in Britain.* London: George Allen and Unwin

Russell, J. K. (1970). 'Pregnancy in the young teenager.' *Practitioner* **204**, 401–405

Rutter, M. (1966). *Children of Sick Parents. An Environmental and Psychiatric Study.* London: Oxford University Press

Rutter, M. (1971). 'Parent–child separation: Psychological effects on the children.' *J. child Psychol. Psychiat.* **12**, 233–260

Sadoff, R. (1971). 'Clinical measure of enforced group psychotherapy (Abstract).' American Psychiatric Association Meetings. Washington

Salmon, M. A. (1971). 'The spectrum of abuse in the battered child syndrome.' *Injury* **2**, 211–217

Sattes, H. (1972). 'Psychopathy.' In *Encyclopaedia of Psychology,* Ed. by H. J. Eysenck, W. A. Arnold and R. Meili, London: Research Press

Sattin, D. B. and Miller, J. K. (1971). 'The ecology of child abuse in a military community.' *Am. J. Orthopsychiat.* **41**, 675–678

Schaffer, H. R. (1974). Personal communication

Schaffer, H. R., Greenwood, A. and Parry, M. H. (1972). 'The onset of wariness.' *Child Dev.* **43**, 165–175

Schaffer, H. R. and Schaffer, E. B. (1968). 'Child care and the family. A study of short term admission to care.' *Occasional Papers on Social Administration,* No. 25. London: Bell and Sons

Schloesser, P. T. (1964). 'The abused child.' *Bull. Menninger Clin.* **28**, 260–268

Schneider, C., Helfer, R. E. and Pollock, C. (1972). 'The predictive questionnaire. A preliminary report.' In *Helping the Battered Child and His Family.* Ed. by C. H. Kempe and R. E. Helfer. Philadelphia and Toronto: J. B. Lippincott

Scott, P. D. (1973). 'Fatal battered baby cases.' Med. *Sci. Law* **13**, 197–206

Sears, R. R., Maccoby, E. E. and Levin, H. H. (1957). *Patterns of Child Rearing.* New York, Evanston and London: Harper and Row

Shaw, A. (1964). 'The surgeon and the battered child.' *Surgery Gynec. Obstet.* **119**, 355

Siker, E. (1967). 'First years' experience in Connecticut with a child abuse law.' *Conn. Hlth Bull.* **81**, 53–59

Silber, D. L. and Bell, W. E. (1971). 'The neurologist and the physically abused child.' *Neurology* **21**, 991–999

Silver, L. B. (1968). 'Child abuse syndrome: A review.' *Med. Times* **96**, 803–820

Silver, L. B. Barton, W. and Dublin, C. C. (1967). 'Child abuse laws – are they enough?' *J. Am. med. Ass.* **199**, 65–68

Silver, L. B. Dublin, C. C. and Lourie, R. S. (1969*a*). 'Child abuse syndrome: The "gray areas" in establishing a diagnosis.' *Pediatrics* **44**, 594–600

Silver, L. B., Dublin, C. C. and Lourie, R. S. (1969*b*). 'Does violence breed violence? Contributions from a study of the child abuse syndrome.' *Am. J. Psychiat.* **126**, 404–407

Silver, H. K. and Finkelstein, M. (1967). 'Deprivation dwarfism.' *J. Pediat.* **70**, 317–324

Silverman, F. N. (1953). 'The roentgen manifestations of unrecognized skeletal trauma in infants.' *Am. J. Roentgen. rad. Ther. nucl. Med.* **69**, 413–426

Silverman, F. N. (1968). 'Radiologic aspects of the battered child syndrome.' In *The Battered Child,* Ed. by R. E. Helfer and C. H. Kempe. Chicago: University of Chicago Press

Silverman, F. N. (1972). 'Unrecognized trauma in infants: The battered child syndrome of Ambroise Tardieu.' *Radiology* **104**, 337–353

Simons, B. and Downs, E. F. (1968). 'Medical reporting of child abuse. Patterns, problems and accomplishments.' *N. Y. St. J. Med.* **68**, 2324–2330

Simons, B., Downs, E. F., Hurster, M. M. and Archer, M. (1966). Child abuse: Epidemiologic study of medically reported cases.' *N. Y. St. J. Med.* **66**, 2783–2788

Simpson, K. (1965). 'Battered babies: Conviction for murder.' *Br. med. J.* **I**, 393

Simpson, K. (1967). 'The battered baby problem.' *R. Soc. Hlth J.* **87**, 168–170

Simpson, K. (1968). 'The battered baby problem.' *S. Afr. med. J.* **42**, 661–663

Skinner, A. E. and Castle, R. L. (1969). *Seventy-eight battered Children: A Retrospective Study:* London: National Society for the Prevention of Cruelty to Children

Slavson, S. R. (1955). 'Criteria for selection and rejection of patients for various kinds of group therapy.' *Int. J. Grp. Psychother.* **5**, 3–30

Smith, M. J. (1950). 'Subdural hematoma with multiple fractures.' *Am. J. Roentgen.* **6**, 342–344

Smith, S. M. (1972). 'Child abuse syndrome.' *Br. med. J.* **III**, 666–670

Smith, S. M. (1973). 'Child injury intensive monitoring system.' *Br. med. J.* **III**, 593–594

Smith, S. M. and Hanson, R. (1972). 'Failure to thrive and anorexia nervosa.'

Postgrad. med. J. **48**, 382–384

Smith, S. M. and Hanson, R. (1974). 'One hundred and thirty-four battered children: A medical and psychological study.' *Br. med. J.* **III**, 666–670

Smith, S. M., Hanson, R. and Noble, S. (1973). 'Parents of battered babies: A controlled study.' *Br. med. J.* **IV**, 388–391

Smith, S. M., Hanson, R. and Noble, S. (1974). 'Social aspects of the battered baby syndrome.' *Br. J. Psychiat.* **125**, 568–582

Smith, S. M., Honigsberger, L. and Smith, C. A. (1973). 'EEG and personality factors in baby batterers.' *Br. med. J.* **II**, 20–22

Smith, S. M. and Noble, S. (1973). 'Battered children and their parents.' *New Soc.* **26**, 393–395

Snedecor, S. T., Knapp, R. E. and Wilson, H. B. (1935). 'Traumatic ossifying periostitis of the newborn.' *Surgery, Gynec. Obstet.* **61**, 385–387

Snedeker, L. (1962). 'Traumatization of children.' *New Engl. J. Med.* **267**, 572

Social Trends (1972). No. 3. Central Statistics Office, H.M.S.O.

Soddy, K. (1964). 'The unwanted child.' *J. fam. Welf.* **11**, 39–52

Spinetta, J. J. and Rigler, D. (1972). 'The child abusing parent: A psychological review.' *Psychol. Bull.* **77**, 296–304

Stafford-Clark, D. and Taylor, F. H. (1949). 'Clinical and electro-encephalographic studies of prisoners charged with murder.' *J. Neurol., Neurosurg. Psychiat.* **12**, 325–330

State of Illinois (1966). A survey of the first year: Illinois child abuse act. Department of Children and Family Services

State of Maryland (1968). Incidents of suspected child abuse, January–June, 1967. Research Report No. 4. Department of Public Welfare

Steele, B. F. (1966). Proceedings of conference on patterns of parental behaviour leading to physical abuse of children. University of Colorado School of Medicine. Unpublished

Steele, B. F. and Pollock, C. B. (1968). 'A psychiatric study of parents who abuse infants and small children. In *The Battered Child,* Ed. by R. E. Helfer and C. H. Kempe. Chicago: University of Chicago Press

Stengel, E. (1964). *Suicide and Attempted Suicide.* Harmondsworth, Middlesex: Penguin Books

Stern, E. S. (1948). 'The medea complex: The mother's homicidal wishes to her child.' *J. ment. Sci.* **94**, 321–331

Stone, N. H., Rinaldo, L., Humphrey, C. R. and Brown, R. H. (1970). 'Child abuse by burning.' *Surg. Clins N. Am.* **50**, 1419–1424

Storey, B. (1964). 'The battered child.' *Med. J. Aust.* **II**. 789–791

Sumner, W. G. (1906). Folways, Boston. Ginn

Sussman, S. J. (1968). 'Skin manifestations of the battered child syndrome.' *J. Pediat.* **72**, 99–101

Swischuk, L. E. (1969). 'Spine and spinal cord trauma in the battered child syndrome.' *Radiology* **92**, 733–738

Tabibian, Y. (1969). 'Les enfants victimes de sévices.' *Méd. Hyg.* **27**, 272–273

Talukder, M. Q. K. and Dawson, K. P. (1974). 'Nutritional marasmus in an affluent society.' *Practitioner* **212**, 359–362

Tardieu, A. (1860). 'Etude médico-legale sur les services et mauvais traitments exerces sur des enfants.' *Hyg. publ. Méd. Lég.* **13**, 361–398

Taylor, S. and Chave, S. (1964). *Mental Health and Environment.* London: Longmans, Green and Co

Ten Bensel, R. W. (1963). 'The battered child syndrome.' *Minn. Med.* **46**, 977–982

Ten Have, R. (1965). 'A preventative approach to problems of child abuse and neglect.' *Mich. Med.* **64**, 645–649

Touloukian, R. J. (1968). 'Abdominal visceral injuries in battered children.' *Pediatrics* **42**, 642–646

Tunbridge Wells Study Group on Non-Accidental Injury to Children (1973). Report and resolutions. (Compiled by A. White Franklin.) Medical Education and Information Unit of the Spastics Society. Department of Health and Social Security.

Tuteur, W. and Glotzer, (1966). 'Further observations on murdering mothers.' *J. forens. Sci.* **11**, 373–383

United States Department of Health, Education and Welfare. (1969). Bibliography on the battered child. Washington D. C. United States Government Printing Office.

Van Stolk, M. (1972). *The Battered Child in Canada.* Toronto: McCleland and Stewart

Vazquez, H. J. and Turner, M. (1951). 'Epilepsia en flexion generalizada.' *Archos Argent. Pediat.* **35**, 111–141

Vesterdal, J. (1972). 'The battered child syndrome.' *Annls Nestlé* **27**, 5–12

Wadsworth, M. (1974). National Survey of Health and Development. Personal communication. Unpublished data.

Walker, N. (1968). *Crime and Insanity in England. Vol. I. The Historical Perspective.* Edinburgh: Edinburgh University Press

Walker, N. (1971). *Crimes, Courts and Figures. An Introduction to Criminal Statistics.* Harmondsworth, Middlesex: Penguin Books

Walker, M. and McCabe, S. (1973). *Crime and Insanity in England. Vol. II. New Solutions and New Problems.* Edinburgh: Edinburgh University Press

Walton, H. J. and Presly, A. S. (1973). 'Abnormal personality.' *Br. J. Psychiat.* **122**, 259–268

Wasserman, S. (1967). 'The abused parent of the abused child.' *Children* **14**, 175–179

Wechsler, D. (1955). *Manual for the Wechsler Adult Intelligence Scale.* New York: The Psychological Corporation

Wedge, P. and Prosser, H. (1973). *Born to Fail.* London: Arrow Books

Weir, S. (1970). A study of unmarried mothers and their children in Scotland. Scottish Health Service Studies No. 13. Scottish Home and Health Department, Edinburgh

Weiss, R. S. (1970). 'Marriage and the family in the near future.' In *The Family and its Future* (Ciba Foundation Symposium), Ed. by K. Elliot. London: Churchill

Werner, O. H. (1917). *The Unmarried Mother in German Literature.* New York: Columbia University Press

West, W. J. (1841). 'On a peculiar form of infantile convulsions?' *Lancet* **1**, 724

West, S. (1888). 'Acute periosteal swellings in several young infants of the same family, probably rickety in nature.' *Br. med. J.* **I**, 856–857

West, D. J. and Farrington, D. P. (1973). *Who Becomes Delinquent?* (Second Report of the Cambridge Study in Delinquent Development). London: Heinemann Educational Books

Weston, W. J. (1957). 'Metaphyseal fractures in infancy.' *J. Bone Jt Surg.* **39**, 694–700

Weston, J. T. (1968). 'The pathology of child abuse.' In *The Battered Child,* Ed. by R. E. Helfer and C. H. Kempe. Chicago: University of Chicago Press

White Franklin, A. (Editor). (1975). *Concerning Child Abuse.* (Papers presented by the Tunbridge Wells Study Group on non-accidental injury to children). London: Churchill-Livingstone

Whitten, C. F., Pettit, M. G. and Fischoff, J. (1969). 'Evidence that growth failure from maternal deprivation is secondary to undereating.' *J. Am. med. Ass.* **209**, 1675–1682

Williams, A. E. (1966). *Barnardo of Stepney: The Father of Nobody's Children.* London: George, Allen and Unwin

Williams, D. (1941). 'The significance of an abnormal electro-encephalogram. *J. Neurol. Psychiat.* **4**, 257–268

Willmott, P. and Young, M. (1960). *Family and Class in a London Suburb.* London: Routledge and Kegan Paul

Winick, M. (1969). 'Malnutrition and brain development.' *J. Pediat.* **74**, 667–679

Woolley, P. V., Jr. and Evans, W. A., Jr. (1955). 'Significance of skeletal lesions in infants resembling those of traumatic origin.' *J. Am. med. Ass.* **158**, 539–543

World Health Organization (1968). *International Classification of Diseases.* Geneva: W.H.O.

Young, L. (1964). *Wednesday's Children: A Study of Child Neglect and Abuse.* New York: McGraw-Hill

Zalba, S. R. (1966). 'The abused child – I. A survey of the problem.' *Social Work*, **11**, 3–16

Zalba, S. R. (1967). 'The abused child – II. A typology for classification and treatment.' *Social Work* **12**, 70–79

Zuckerman, P. N. and Lubin, B. (1965). *A preliminary Manual for Multiple Affect Adjective Check List.* Unpublished

Index